Pancreatic Cystic Neoplasms

George H. Sakorafas
Vassileios Smyrniotis • Michael G. Sarr
Editors

Pancreatic Cystic Neoplasms

From Imaging to Differential Diagnosis and Management

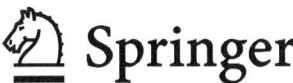 Springer

Editors
George H. Sakorafas, MD
4th Dept Surgery
ATTIKON University Hospital
Athens
Greece

Michael G. Sarr, MD
Department of Surgery
Mayo Clinic
Rochester, Minnesota
USA

Vassileios Smyrniotis, MD
Surgery
ATTIKON University Hospital, Athens
Greece
Athens
Attiki
Greece

ISBN 978-88-470-5707-4   ISBN 978-88-470-5708-1   (eBook)
DOI 10.1007/978-88-470-5708-1
Springer Milan Heidelberg New York Dordrecht London

Library of Congress Control Number: 2014956531

Printed on acid-free paper

Springer is part of Springer Science+Business Media (www.springer.com)

To Greek surgeons practicing surgery in hard times

Preface

It is with great delight that we present this monograph devoted to pancreatic cystic neoplasms. This work summarizes our knowledge regarding biologic behavior, histopathology, current diagnostic approach, and optimal treatment of these increasingly recognized pancreatic lesions. The up-to-date treatise is the result of an increased and long-standing interest of the editors in pancreatic surgery and specifically in the operative and nonoperative management of pancreatic cystic neoplasms. We would like to express our appreciation to our co-authors who have contributed two very important chapters (on histopathology and imaging) and we wish to recognize these and thank them for their dedication and commitment. We would also like to thank the editorial and production team at Springer and Mrs. Deborah Frank who have been instrumental in making this edition a reality.

Athens, Greece   George H. Sakorafas
Athens, Attiki, Greece   Vassileios Smyrniotis
Rochester, MN, USA   Michael G. Sarr

Contents

Contributors

Rondell P.D. Graham Division of Anatomic Pathology, Department of Laboratory Medicine and Pathology, Mayo Clinic, Rochester, MN, USA

Dimitrios Kechagias CT and MRI Department, Hygeia Hospital, Athens, Greece

Fotios Laspas CT and MRI Department, Hygeia Hospital, Athens, Greece

George H. Sakorafas Department of Surgical Oncology, Saint Savvas Cancer Hospital, Athens, Greece

Michael G. Sarr Department of Surgery, Mayo Clinic, Rochester, MN, USA

Thomas C. Smyrk Division of Anatomic Pathology, Department of Laboratory Medicine and Pathology, Mayo Clinic, Rochester, MN, USA

Vassileios Smyrniotis 4th Department of Surgery, Attikon University Hospital, Athens, Greece

Introduction to Pancreatic Cystic Neoplasms

George H. Sakorafas, Vassileios Smyrniotis, and Michael G. Sarr

Over the last three decades, pancreatic cystic neoplasms (PCNs) are being appreciated and recognized with increasing frequency, primarily as a result of increased awareness of these neoplasms and their natural history and the widespread availability and extensive use of ever improving modalities of cross-sectional imaging [1]. Commonly, PCNs are diagnosed incidentally during investigation for often unrelated and nonspecific abdominal complaints using state-of-the art abdominal imaging. The use of the term PCN encompasses a histologically heterogenous group of neoplasms with a wide spectrum of biologic behavior, ranging from completely benign to potentially malignant, to *carcinoma* in situ, to frankly invasive and malignant [2]. In 1978, Compagno and Oertel were the first to recognize the crucial distinction between the serous and the mucinous cystic neoplasms of the pancreas by explaining the importance of identifying the mucinous neoplasms because of their overt or latent malignant potential [3, 4]. Since then, the interest in PCNs increased markedly, especially so with the recognition of the importance and prevalence of intraductal papillary mucinous neoplasms (IPMNs).

Nowadays, PCNs represent a common and often difficult problem in clinical practice, because of the increase in their detection in asymptomatic patients and our still immature understanding of some aspects of their biologic behavior. This

G.H. Sakorafas, MD (✉)
Department of Surgical Oncology, Saint Savvas Cancer Hospital,
Arkadias 19-21, Athens 11526, Greece
e-mail: georgesakorafas@yahoo.com

V. Smyrniotis, MD
4th Department of Surgery, Attikon University Hospital, Chanioti 22, Athens 15452, Greece
e-mail: vsmyrniotis@hotmail.com

M.G. Sarr, MD
J C Masson Professor of Surgery, Department of Surgery, Mayo Clinic
Rochester, MN 55902, USA
e-mail: sarr.michel@mayo.edu

© Springer-Verlag Italia 2015
G.H. Sakorafas et al. (eds.), *Pancreatic Cystic Neoplasms:*
From Imaging to Differential Diagnosis and Management,
DOI 10.1007/978-88-470-5708-1_1

increase in recognition – in conjunction with their important differences regarding their biologic behavior – has led to a marked focus of interest in these neoplasms by surgeons, pathologists, gastroenterologists, radiologists, and oncologists alike. Management of patients with PCNs can be challenging and varies considerably among the various subtypes of PCNs. Accurate classification of pancreatic cystic lesions is of crucial importance, because premalignant lesions will require resection and/or surveillance, malignant lesions require resection, and others that are benign or indolent can be observed. Appropriate classification and therapeutic decision-making are based mainly on the presenting symptoms and radiologic findings, often without actual histologic tissue. Suspicious features indicating underlying malignancy or malignant potential should be identified and are of particular importance for selecting appropriate treatment. The risk of overtreatment (unnecessary pancreatectomy) should be balanced carefully with the risk of undertreatment (missing the opportunity to cure a potentially curable malignant or premalignant disease) [5]. Unfortunately, despite the availability of many sophisticated diagnostic tools, accurate preoperative diagnosis is often not possible [6]; this uncertainty emphasizes the problems and challenges in treating patients with PCNs [7]. The aim of this monograph is to summarize and critically analyze currently available data regarding optimal management of these fascinating PCNs.

References

1. Gajoux S, Brennan MF, Gonen M, et al. Cystic lesions of the pancreas: changes in the presentation and management of 1,424 patients at a single institution over a 15-year time period. J Am Coll Surg. 2011;212:590–600.
2. Brugge WR, Lauwers GY, Sahani D, Fernandez-del Castillo C, Warshaw AL. Cystic neoplasms of the pancreas. N Engl J Med. 2004;351:1218–26.
3. Compagno J, Oertel JE. Microcystic adenomas of the pancreas (glycogen-rich cystadenomas): a clinicopathologic study of 34 cases. Am J Clin Pathol. 1978;69:289–98.
4. Compagno J, Oertel JE. Mucinous cystic neoplasms of the pancreas with overt and latent malignancy (cystadenocarcinomas and cystadenomas): a clinicopathologic study of 41 cases. Am J Clin Pathol. 1978;69:573–80.
5. Lennon AM, Wolfgang C. Cystic neoplasms of the pancreas. J Gastrointest Surg. 2013;17:645–53.
6. Correa-Gallego C, Ferrone CR, Thayer SP, et al. Incidental pancreatic cysts: do we really know what we are watching? Pancreatology. 2010;10:144–50.
7. Cho CS, Russ AJ, Loeffler AG, et al. Preoperative classification of pancreatic cystic neoplasms: the clinical significance of diagnostic inaccuracy. Ann Surg Oncol. 2013. doi:10.1245/s10434-013-2986-6.

George H. Sakorafas, Vassileios Smyrniotis,
and Michael G. Sarr

Asymptomatic cystic lesions of the pancreas are not uncommon; indeed, their incidence is about 1 in 100 hospitalized patients [1]. These cystic lesions represent a diverse spectrum of disease, encompassing traumatic, infectious, congenital, or neoplastic etiologies (Table 2.1). The incidence of cystic lesions of the pancreas increases with age [2, 3] and depends on the method used for their detection. In an autopsy study, Kimura et al. found that the incidence of pancreatic cystic lesions of all types was 24 % and that these lesions were distributed equally throughout the pancreas [2]. In a population of 24,039 patients undergoing computed tomography (CT) or magnetic resonance imaging (MRI) during the period 1995–2002, Spinelli et al. identified pancreatic "cysts" in 1.2 % of patients, and 0.7 % of the sample had no history of pancreatitis [4]. Using the newer, multi-detector CT, unexpected, unrelated, and incidental pancreatic "cysts" were identified with a prevalence of 2.6 % [5]. The prevalence is even greater when MRI is used, ranging from 2.4 to 13.5 % [6]. Zhang et al. [7] estimated that the prevalence of pancreatic "cysts" (many being <1 cm) in patients undergoing MRI for non-pancreatic diseases was nearly 20 %. Girometti et al. reported the prevalence of pancreatic "cysts" to be 44.7 % in patients undergoing MRCP for non-pancreatic indications [8]. There is evidence that many of these pancreatic cystic lesions are unrecognized and have been underdiagnosed, because a substantial percentage (up to 70 %!) of pancreatic cystic lesions are not

G.H. Sakorafas, MD (✉)
Department of Surgical Oncology, Saint Savvas Cancer Hospital,
Arkadias 19-21, Athens 11526, Greece
e-mail: georgesakorafas@yahoo.com

V. Smyrniotis, MD
4th Department of Surgery, Attikon University Hospital, Chanioti 22, Athens 15452, Greece
e-mail: vsmyrniotis@hotmail.com

M.G. Sarr, MD
Department of Surgery, Mayo Clinic, 200 First Street SW, Rochester, MN 55905, USA
e-mail: sarr.michael@mayo.edu

© Springer-Verlag Italia 2015
G.H. Sakorafas et al. (eds.), *Pancreatic Cystic Neoplasms:
From Imaging to Differential Diagnosis and Management*,
DOI 10.1007/978-88-470-5708-1_2

Table 2.1 Cystic lesions of the pancreas

Cystic neoplasms
Serous cystic neoplasms (SCNs)
Mucinous cystic neoplasms (MCNs)
Intraductal papillary mucinous neoplasms (IPMNs)
Uncommon cystic neoplasms
Solid pseudopapillary neoplasm
Cystic neuroendocrine neoplasms (functional and nonfunctional)
Acinar cell cystadenocarcinoma
Angiomatous neoplasm (angioma, lymphangioma, hemangioendothelioma)
Cystic teratoma
Cystic choriocarcinoma
Acquired cystic lesions
Pancreatic pseudocyst
Pancreatic pseudopseudocyst (inflammatory exudative collection)
Postinflammatory cystic fluid collection
Acute necrotic collection
Walled-off necrosis
Echinococcal (hydatid) cyst
Parasitic cysts
Taenia solium cyst
Congenital cysts (true cysts)
True cysts (rare primary pancreatic cyst)
Pancreatic cysts associated with polycystic disease of the kidneys
Polycystic disease of the pancreas without related anomalies
Pancreatic macrocysts associated with cystic fibrosis
Polycystic disease of the pancreas associated with cerebellar neoplasms and retinal angiomata (von Hippel-Lindau disease)
Enterogenous cysts (duplication cysts)
Endometriosis dermoid cysts

Modified from Sakorafas et al. [36]

reported in the original radiology report [6]. The increasing prevalence of incidentally diagnosed pancreatic cystic lesions has also been reported in the surgical literature, where an increase by 28 % over 33 years has been documented [9].

Increased awareness and improved sensitivity of imaging is associated not only with increasing detection rates but also with decreasing lesion size [10–13]. These factors only increase the clinical challenges involved in determining which patients require either more investigation, surveillance, or resection. Ferrone et al. compared data for the periods 1997–2002 and 2004–2007 and noted that the proportion of asymptomatic patients being referred to PCNs increased from 36 to 71 %; interestingly, the proportion undergoing resection decreased from 80 to 50 % [11]. Recently, it has been reported that the median size of cystic lesions of the pancreas in patients being referred for lesions sent for evaluation halved from 4 to 2 cm over the last 5-year period [14, 15]. Ferrone and colleagues reported a similar decrease in the size of lesions referred from 3.3 to 2.7 cm [11].

PCNs were considered previously to be a rare entity, being identified during transabdominal ultrasonography in 0.2 % of studies [16]. Currently, PCNs have become a surprisingly common clinical problem, accounting for 10–15 % of all cystic lesions of the pancreas [17, 18]. The vast majority (~90 %) of PCNs are serous cystic neoplasms (SCNs), primary mucinous cystic neoplasms of the pancreas (MCNs), or IPMN [3, 19, 20] (Tables 2.1 and 2.2). Other rare types of PCNs (solid pseudopapillary neoplasms, cystic neuroendocrine neoplasms, etc.) account for about 10 % of all cases of PCNs.

SCNs account for over 30 % of PCNs and for 1 % of non-endocrine pancreatic neoplasms. SCNs arise anywhere in the pancreas, with most cases occurring in the pancreatic head [21, 23] (Table 2.2). In a multicenter study from Japan, SCNs were located in the pancreatic head, body, tail, and uncinate process in 39, 35, 22, and 3 % of patients, respectively [22]. SCNs typically occur in women over the age of 60, with a female to male ratio of 70:30 [24, 25]. In a study from the Massachusetts General Hospital, Tseng et al. [25] reviewed 106 patients with SCNs of the pancreas, 75 % of whom were females. Mean age at presentation was 62 years, but the mean age of males was >7 years older than that of females, and males had larger tumors at presentation, suggesting a delay in diagnosis in men [25].

MCNs occur almost exclusively (>95 %) in middle-aged/perimenopausal females [26–28]. Literature in the past suggested a much more common prevalence in men than we appreciate currently; in retrospect, most of these lesions in men were IPMNs and not MCNs. This topic will be discussed below. The incidence of MCNs peaks in the fifth decade of life [29, 30]. MCNs arise in the body and tail of the pancreas in approximately 95 % of patients [23].

IPMNs represent an increasingly recognized neoplasm. In a large, retrospective study of resected pancreatic cystic lesions, IPMNs were the most commonly resected cystic lesion accounting for about 2 % of cases [9]. IPMNs occur slightly more commonly in men between the ages of 50 and 80 (older than patients with MCNs) [8, 31]. While IPMNs usually arise in the head of the pancreas, they can occur anywhere in the pancreas, as well as arising in multiple locations in 20–30 % of cases when looked for with diligence [23]. In 5–10 % of patients, they may involve the pancreas diffusely as multicentric IPMN [32]. IPMNs are classified as main duct IPMN, branch duct IPMN arising only in side branches off the main pancreatic duct, or mixed IPMN arising in both the main duct and the side branches. While main duct IPMNs (see below) are more common in men, branch duct IPMNs occur more commonly in women [33].

The more unusual PCNs represent about 10 % of all PCNs. Solid pseudopapillary neoplasms (SPNs) occur almost exclusively (~90 %) in young women (21–33 years of age) and account for 1–3.5 % of PCNs [9, 34, 35]; SPNs may occur anywhere throughout the pancreas. Cystic degeneration of ductal adenocarcinoma accounts for 0.8 % of all PCNs, while cystic pancreatic neuroendocrine neoplasms account for about 7.3 % of all PCNs and may be associated with MEN1 syndrome.

Table 2.2 Features of PPNCs: Clinical and imaging

	Pseudocyst	SCN	MCN	IPMN	SPPT	Lymphoepithelial cyst
Clinical						
Sex ratio (M/F)	1:1	1:3–4	1:9	1–2:1	1:10	4:1
Age, range (year)	30–50	60–80	30–50	60–80	15–40	30–80
Prior pancreatopathy	Pancreatitis	None	None	May have symptoms of acute or more commonly chronic pancreatitis	None	None
Findings on cross-sectional imaging						
Location in pancreas	Most commonly neck/body	Head>body/tail	Body/tail>>head	Head>body/tail	Evenly distributed	Most commonly body/tail
Uni-/multicentric	Unicentric	Unicentric	Unicentric	Unicentric, but can be multicentric	Unicentric	Unicentric
Characteristics of lesions	Uni-/multiloculated rounded shape macrocysts, pericystic inflammation reaction, findings of pancreatitis	Multiple, small (<2 cm) microcysts; rarely a unilocular macrocyst; characteristic central stellate calcification (~30 %)	Unilocular or multiloculated macrocysts >2 cm, smooth external contour	Irregular, polycystic mass with dilation of main and/or branch ducts	Large, encapsulated solid/cystic mass, "cystic" areas	Encapsulated, uni- or more commonly multiloculated cyst in and/or around the gland

Findings suggestive of malignancy	None	Rare <1 % serous cystadenocarcinoma, invasive and/or metastatic lesions	Eggshell calcification, solid component, or mural nodule	Main duct (dilation, >1 cm), branch duct lesion (>3 cm with solid component), mural nodules; systemic symptoms – weight loss, jaundice	Metastatic disease (rare, usually present at diagnosis)	None
Findings on ERCP/MRCP						
Communication of cystic area with pancreatic duct	Present	Absent	Absent	Present. Main or side branch dilation	Absent	Absent
Findings on EUS						
	Unilocular macrocystic lesion, internal debris, thick wall, pericystic reaction	Microcystic, honeycombed, rarely macrocystic, no pericystic reaction	Macrocystic, septae within the "cyst," no pericystic reaction	Dilated pancreatic duct (main duct or side branches)	Mixed solid and cystic lesion	Thin-walled, heterogeneous, subtle posterior enhancement

Modified from Sakorafas et al. [36]

Other much more rare PCNs have been reported in the literature usually as case reports and include cystic acinar cell carcinomas, teratomas, serous cystadenocarcinomas, and a few others.

References

1. Khalid A, Brugge W. ACG practice guidelines for the diagnosis and management of neoplastic pancreatic cysts. Am J Gastroenterol. 2007;102:2339–49.
2. Kimura W, Nagai H, Kuroda A, Muto T, Esaki Y. Analysis of small cystic lesions of the pancreas. Int J Pancreatol. 1995;18:197–206.
3. Kosmahl M, Pauser U, Peters K, Sipos B, Lüttges J, Kremer B, et al. Cystic neoplasms of the pancreas and tumor-like lesions with cystic features: a review of 418 cases and a classification proposal. Virchows Arch. 2004;445:168–78.
4. Spinelli KS, Fromwiller TE, Daniel RA, Kiely JM, Nakeen A, Komorowski RA, et al. Cystic pancreatic neoplasms: observe or operate. Ann Surg. 2004;239:651–7.
5. Laffan TA, Horton KM, Klein AP, Berlanstein B, Siegelman SS, Kawamoto S, et al. Prevalence of unsuspected pancreatic cysts on MDCT. AJR Am J Roentgenol. 2008;191:802–7.
6. Lee KS, Sekhar A, Rofsky NM, Pedrosa I. Prevalence of incidental pancreatic cysts in the adult population on MR imaging. Am J Gastroenterol. 2010;105(9):2079–84.
7. Zhang XM, Mitchell DG, Dohke M, Holland GA, Parker L. Pancreatic cysts: depiction on single-shot fast spin-echoMRimages. Radiology. 2002;223:547–53.
8. Girometti R, Intini S, Brondani G, Como G, Londero F, Bresadola F, et al. Incidental pancreatic cysts on 3D turbo spin echo magnetic resonance cholangiopancreatography: prevalence and relation with clinical and imaging features. Abdom Imaging. 2011;36:196–205.
9. Valsangkar N, Morales-Oyarvide V, Thayer S, Ferrone C, Wargo J, Warshaw A, et al. 851 resected cystic tumors of the pancreas: a 33-year experience at the Massachusetts General Hospital. Surgery. 2012;152(3 Suppl 1):S4–12.
10. Allen PJ, D'Angelica M, Gonen M, Jaques DP, Coit DG, Jarnagin WR, et al. A selective approach to the resection of cystic lesions of the pancreas: results from 539 consecutive patients. Ann Surg. 2006;244:572–82.
11. Ferrone CR, Correa-Gallego C, Warshaw AL, Brugge WR, Forcione DG, Thayer SP, et al. Trends in pancreatic cystic neoplasms. Arch Surg. 2009;144:448–54.
12. Correa-Gallego C, Ferrone CR, Thayer SP, Wargo JA, Warshaw AL, Fernandez-del CC. Incidental pancreatic cysts: do we really know what we are watching? Pancreatology. 2010;10:144–50.
13. Gaujoux S, Brennan MF, Gonen M, D'Angelica MI, DeMatteo R, Fong Y, et al. Cystic lesions of the pancreas: changes in the presentation and management of 1424 patients at a single institution over a 15-year time period. J Am Coll Surg. 2011;212:590–600.
14. Gareth M-S, Falk GA, Sricharan C, Matthew Walsh R. Natural history of asymptomatic pancreatic cystic neoplasms. HPB. 2013;15:175–81.
15. Walsh RM, Vogt DP, Henderson JM, Zuccaro G, Vargo J, Dumot J, et al. Natural history of indeterminate pancreatic cysts. Surgery. 2005;138:665–70.
16. Ikeda M, Sato T, Morozumi A, Fujino MA, Yoda Y, Ochiai M, et al. Morphologic changes in the pancreas detected by screening ultrasonography in a mass survey, with special reference to main duct dilatation, cyst formation, and calcification. Pancreas. 1994;9:508–12.
17. Ceppa EP, De la Fuente S, Reddy SK, Stinnett SS, Clary BM, Tyler DS, et al. Defining criteria for selective operative management of pancreatic cystic lesions: does size really matter? J Gastrointest Surg. 2010;14:236–44.
18. Garcea G, Ong SL, Rajesh A, Neal CP, Pollard CA, Berry DP, Dennison AR. Cystic lesions of the pancreas: a diagnostic and management dilemma. Pancreatology. 2008;8:236–51.

19. Sarr MG, Murr M, Smyrk TC, Yeo CJ, Fernandez-del-Castillo C, Hawes RH, et al. Primary cystic neoplasms of the pancreas: neoplastic disorders of emerging importance-current state of the art and unanswered questions. J Gastrointest Surg. 2003;7:417–28.
20. Brugge WR, Lauwers GY, Sahani D, Fernandez-del Castillo C, Warshaw AL. Cystic neoplasms of the pancreas. N Engl J Med. 2004;351:1218–26.
21. Sakorafas GH, Sarr MG. Cystic neoplasms of the pancreas; what a clinician should know. Cancer Treat Rev. 2005;31:507–35.
22. Kimura W, Moriya T, Hanada K, Abe H, Yanagisawa A, Fukushima N, Ohike N, Shimizu M, Hatori T, Fujita N, et al. Multicenter study of SCN of the Japan Pancreas Society: a multiinstitutional study of 172 patients. Pancreas. 2012;41:380–7.
23. Lee LS, Clancy T, Kadiyala V, Suleiman S, Conwell DL. Interdisciplinary management of cystic neoplasms of the pancreas. Gastroenterol Res Pract. 2012;2:1–7.
24. Khashab MA, Shin EJ Amateau S, Canto MI, Hruban RH, Fishman EK, et al. Tumor size and location correlate with behavior of pancreatic serous cystic neoplasms. Am J Gastroenterol. 2011;106:1521–6.
25. Tseng JF, Warshaw AL, Sahani DV, Lauwers GY, Rattner DW, Fernandez-del Castillo C. Serous cystadenoma of the pancreas: tumor growth rates and recommendations for treatment. Ann Surg. 2005;242:413–9.
26. Goh BK, Tan YM, Chung YF, Chow PK, Cheow PC, Wong WK, Ooi LL. A review of mucinous cystic neoplasms of the pancreas defined by ovarian-type stroma: clinicopathological features of 344 patients. World J Surg. 2006;30:2236–45.
27. Goh BK, Tan YM, Kumarasinghe MP, Ooi LL. Mucinous cystic tumor of the pancreas with ovarian-like mesenchymal stroma in a male patient. Dig Dis Sci. 2005;50:2170–7.
28. Zamboni G, Scarpa A, Bogina G, Iacono C, Bassi C, Talamini G, Sessa F, Capella C, Solcia E, Rickaert F, et al. Mucinous cystic tumors of the pancreas: clinicopathological features, prognosis, and relationship to other mucinous cystic tumors. Am J Surg Pathol. 1999;23:410–22.
29. Yoon WJ, Brugge WR. Pancreatic cystic neoplasms: diagnosis and management. Gastroenterol Clin N Am. 2012;41:103–18.
30. Yamao K, Yanagisawa A, Takahashi K, Kimura W, Doi R, Fukushima N, et al. Clinicopathological features and prognosis of mucinous cystic neoplasm with ovarian-type stroma: a multiinstitutional study of the Japan Pancreas Society. Pancreas. 2011;40:67–71.
31. Sohn TA, Yeo CJ, Cameron JL, Hruban RH, Fukushima N, Campbell KA, Lillemoe KD. Intraductal papillary mucinous neoplasms of the pancreas: an updated experience. Ann Surg. 2004;239:788–97.
32. Campbell F, Azadeh B. Cystic neoplasms of the exocrine pancreas. Histopathology. 2008;52(5):539–51.
33. Mohamadnejad M, Eloubeidi MA. Cystic lesions of the pancreas. Arch Iran Med. 2013;16:233–9.
34. Reddy S, Cameron JL, Scudiere J, Hruban RH, Fishman EK, Ahuja N, et al. Surgical management of solid-pseudopapillary neoplasms of the pancreas (Franz or Hamoudi tumors): a large single-institutional series. J Am Coll Surg. 2009;208(5):950–9.
35. Yang F, Fu DL, Jin C, Long J, Yu XJ, Xu J, et al. Clinical experiences of solid pseudopapillary tumors of the pancreas in China. J Gastroenterol Hepatol. 2008;23:1847–51.
36. Sakorafas GH, Smyrniotis V, Reid Lombardo KM, Sarr MG. Primary pancreatic cystic neoplasms revisited. Part I: serous cystic neoplasms. Surg Oncol. 2011;20:e84–92.

Pathology of Pancreatic Cystic Neoplasms

3

Rondell P.D. Graham and Thomas C. Smyrk

3.1 Mucinous Cystic Neoplasm (MCN)

Primary MCN of the pancreas affects females at a ratio of greater than 9:1, can arise in patients less than 50 years old, and is typically located in the body or tail of the pancreas [1, 2]. As a rule, MCN does not communicate with the pancreatic ductal system, although exceptions have been described [3], and a recent series from Japan noted (without additional comment) that 25/138 MCN had a luminal connection to the pancreatic ductal system [4]. Tumor size can range from 1 to 30 cm. MCNs are sometimes unilocular but more often have a complex internal structure comprising thin-walled locules of varying size (Fig. 3.1). As the name implies, the cyst contents tend to be mucinous, although old or recent hemorrhage can alter the color and consistency of the mucus. Palpable or visible solid areas and mural nodules are sometimes present; tumors with such areas are more likely to contain invasive carcinoma, and it is these areas that pathologists sample most assiduously.

The epithelial lining of MCN usually takes the form of a single layer of cuboidal to columnar cells with minimal variation in nuclear size and shape. The bland nuclei are situated near the base of the cell. These minimal changes have been characterized generally as low-grade dysplasia, although some authors have proposed recently that MCN with this morphology should be termed "non-mucinous cystadenoma" and that such lesions have little or no malignant potential [5]. Moderate dysplasia is characterized by increased nuclear pseudostratification and pleomorphism, while high-grade dysplasia has been reserved for those tumors with complex architecture (micropapillary growth, cribriform architecture) and marked

R.P.D. Graham, MBBS (✉) • T.C. Smyrk, MD
Division of Anatomic Pathology, Department of Laboratory Medicine and Pathology,
Mayo Clinic, 200 1st St SW, Rochester, MN, USA
e-mail: graham.rondell@mayo.edu; smyrk.thomas@mayo.edu

© Springer-Verlag Italia 2015
G.H. Sakorafas et al. (eds.), *Pancreatic Cystic Neoplasms:
From Imaging to Differential Diagnosis and Management*,
DOI 10.1007/978-88-470-5708-1_3

Fig. 3.1 Primary MCN of
the pancreas. The outer
contour is smooth, but the
internal structure is complex
with cysts of varying size
separated by thin walls. There
is a solid area at 4 o'clock
which is the most likely place
to find malignancy
(© 1998–2014 Mayo
Foundation for Medical
Education and Research. All
rights reserved)

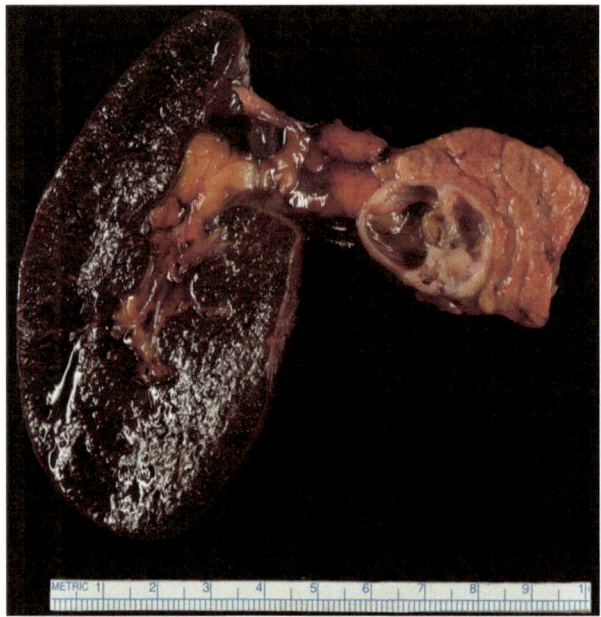

Fig. 3.2 The lining of
MCN. The neoplastic
epithelium is a single layer of
cuboidal cells. The ovarian-
like stroma forms a compact
subepithelial layer populated
by cells with bland, oval
nuclei (© 1998–2014 Mayo
Foundation for Medical
Education and Research. All
rights reserved)

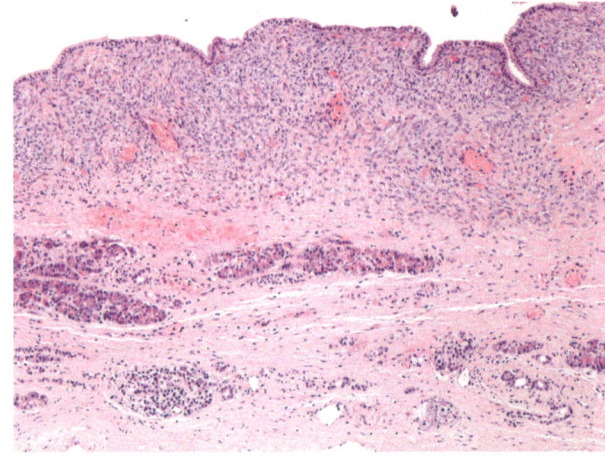

variation in nuclear size and shape. Occasionally, the epithelium in MCN can have
papillary architecture mimicking the lining of intraductal papillary mucinous neoplasm (IPMN). In such cases, other clinicopathologic features (sex, site, absence of
ductal communication, presence of ovarian-like stroma) are clues to the correct
diagnosis. In addition, on occasion the epithelial lining is discontinuous and absent
in areas; therefore, multiple sections may be required to make the diagnosis of MCN
versus a pseudocyst which lacks epithelial lining.

Ovarian-like stroma is a defining feature of MCN (Fig. 3.2). Ovarian stroma
takes the form of bland spindle cells forming a compact layer immediately beneath
the epithelium. The spindle cells are generally positive for estrogen receptor and

progesterone receptor, and the similarity to ovarian stroma is sometimes made even more exact by the finding of inhibin-positive cells, corresponding to luteinized cells of ovarian stroma. As the MCN enlarges, the characteristic stroma may become attenuated and hyalinized; it will not be present in every section. Sufficient sampling will almost always demonstrate this diagnostic criterion, but there will be rare cases that seem to be MCN in every sense save the ovarian-like stroma. In this situation, a descriptive diagnosis may be the best that the pathologist can offer.

MCN is a premalignant lesion. Although the older literature suggested that as many as 30 % of MCNs harbor invasive carcinoma, studies which define MCN specifically and appropriately by the presence of ovarian-like stroma give a prevalence ranging from 3.9 to 13.4 % [4, 6]. When malignancy is present, it almost always resembles conventional ductal carcinoma of the pancreas. Carcinoma in MCN should be further classified as invasive or "minimally invasive" (invasion into ovarian stroma but not beyond the capsule or into the pancreatic parenchyma), because the minimally invasive MCNs are much less likely to recur [7]. Colloid carcinoma traditionally has been considered a possible complication of MCN, but a recent multicenter review comprising 291 MCNs found only one case with even focal mucinous, non-cystic differentiation [6]. Undifferentiated, anaplastic, and sarcomatoid carcinomas have also been described [8, 9]. In cases with invasion, the invasive component is staged based on the criteria set forth by the American Joint Committee on Cancer for ductal pancreatic carcinoma. Given the potentially focal nature of invasion, the MCN should be sampled extensively [10, 11].

Epithelial cells of the MCN are often positive for the mucin core protein MUC5AC with MUC1 expression limited to invasive tumors. MUC2 is typically only positive in rare goblet cells within the tumor [12].

Recently, investigators have identified recurrent genetic alterations in *KRAS*, *GNAS*, and *RNF43* in MCN [13, 14]. These mutations overlap with IPMN and thus are not specific to MCN. Detection of these mutations, however, does support that a cystic mass is neoplastic and together with the appropriate morphology may facilitate diagnosis [13, 14].

3.2   Intraductal Papillary Mucinous Neoplasm (IPMN)

IPMN is a disease of the middle age. It affects males slightly more often than females. IPMN is a mucin-producing neoplasm that arises from the epithelium of the pancreatic ducts and leads to ductal dilation (Fig. 3.3). Based on imaging [15] or gross pathologic examination, the location of ductal involvement can be categorized as main duct, branch duct, or a mixture of both; each category accounts for approximately one-third of resected IPMNs [16–18]. Clinically, this differentiation is an important distinction to make, because main duct (and mixed) IPMNs manifest a much greater risk for malignancy, and therefore, resection is usually advised, while branch duct IPMN can be followed if small, asymptomatic, and free of mural nodules and has no other worrisome features [15] (see Chap. 6). Main duct IPMN is seen most commonly in the head of the pancreas, though about a third of IPMNs arise in the body or tail of the organ; some proximal-based IPMNs produce diffuse

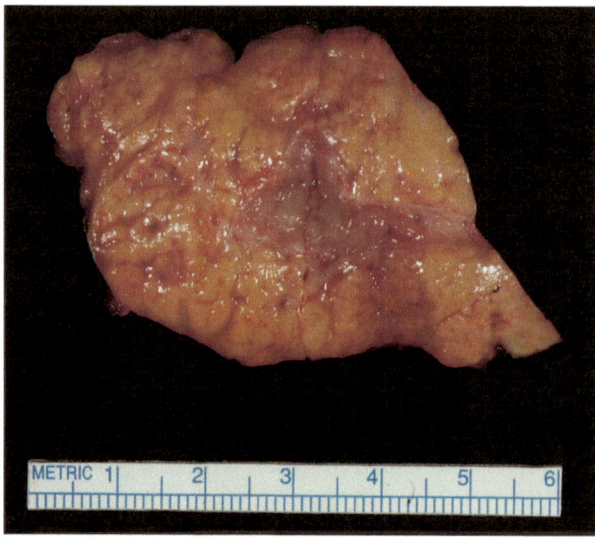

Fig. 3.3 IPMN dilating the main pancreatic duct and extending into several side branches (© 1998–2014 Mayo Foundation for Medical Education and Research. All rights reserved)

duct ectasia involving the entire pancreas. Branch duct IPMN is most often found in the head or uncinate process of the pancreas, but with high-resolution imaging, other smaller branch duct IPMNs are often seen as well.

Microscopically, IPMNs are lined by mucin-producing cells which may be arranged in a flat layer but more often present as papillary projections. The epithelial cells may recapitulate a gastric foveolar, intestinal, pancreaticobiliary, or oncocytic lining (Fig. 3.4). The intestinal form of epithelium represents the most common type of epithelium seen in IPMNs. Intestinal-type IPMNs feature long, slender papillae lined by tall columnar cells with oval nuclei. MUC2 and CDX2 label the neoplastic cells. The intestinal-type IPMNs may be associated with malignant transformation; the cancers that arise in this setting are mucinous (colloid) carcinomas (Fig. 3.5). The gastric foveolar type of epithelium common in branch duct IPMNs has a much less risk of malignant transformation. This type of epithelium appears very bland with abundant mucin and regularly oriented, basal nuclei. These neoplastic cells express MUC5AC. The pancreatobiliary-type IPMN has complex papillae lined by cuboidal cells which stain positive for MUC1. This type of IMPN has the greatest risk for malignant transformation, and the cancer that arises in this background is a ductal adenocarcinoma. Lastly, the oncocytic type of epithelium is characterized by cells with abundant, granular eosinophilic cytoplasm, reflecting their large numbers of mitochondria. The neoplasm forms complex papillae or solid sheets with occasional admixed goblet cells.

The epithelium of all types of IPMN is classified histopathologically according to the degree of dysplasia [19, 20]. Briefly, low-grade dysplasia refers to retained nuclear polarity, minimal variation of nuclear shape, and slight nuclear enlargement. High-grade dysplasia is characterized by architectural complexity, loss of nuclear polarity, marked nuclear pleomorphism, and prominent irregularity (Fig. 3.6). Moderate dysplasia is intermediate between these two categories [20].

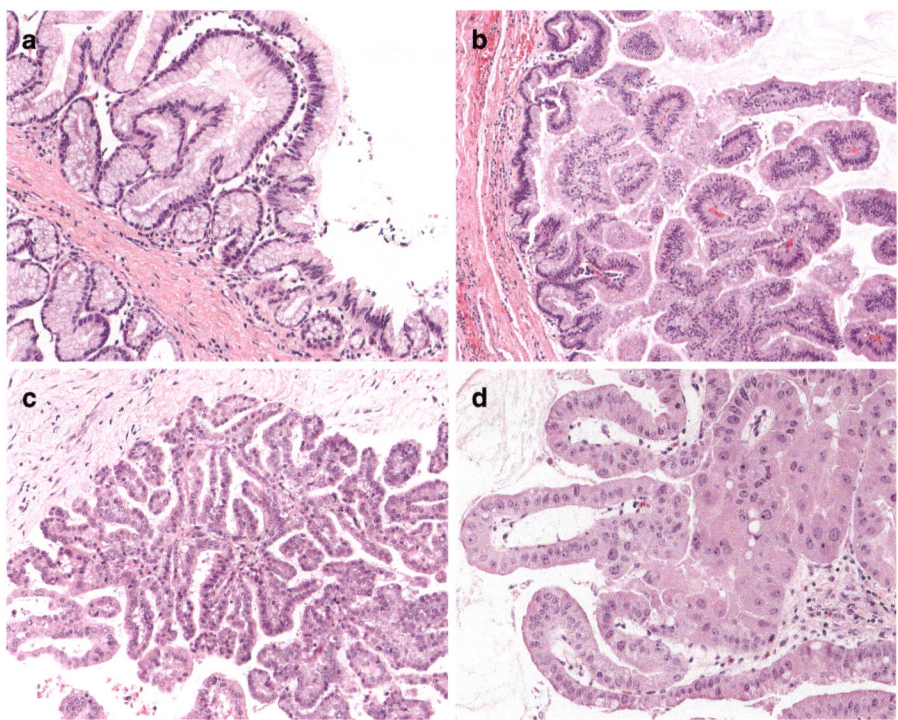

Fig. 3.4 Subtypes of IPMN. (**a**) Gastric-type lining has bland cells with abundant mucin and round, basally oriented nuclei. (**b**) Intestinal-type epithelium features tall columnar cells with oval, often pseudostratified nuclei. (**c**) The cuboidal cells of pancreatobiliary-type lining. Nuclei are round and the nucleus/cytoplasm ratio is greater than in the other cell types. (**d**) Oncocytic IPMN has large cuboidal cells with abundant granular cytoplasm (© 1998–2014 Mayo Foundation for Medical Education and Research. All rights reserved)

Fig. 3.5 Colloid carcinoma (also known as mucinous non-cystic carcinoma) producing abundant extracellular mucin associated with an intestinal-type IPMN at the *right* (© 1998–2014 Mayo Foundation for Medical Education and Research. All rights reserved)

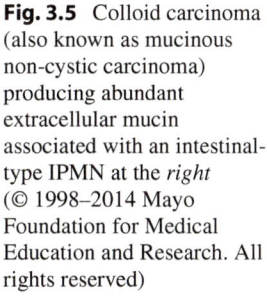

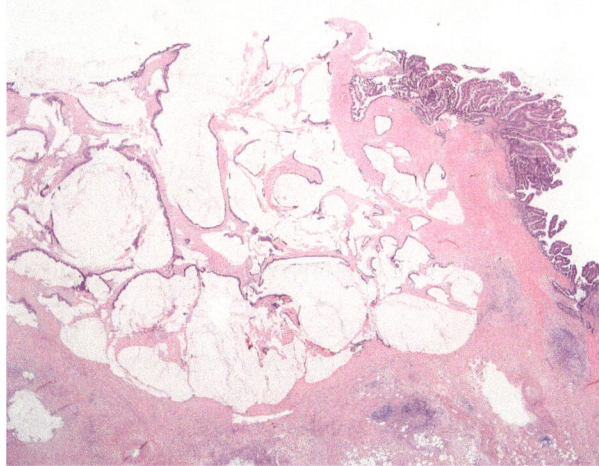

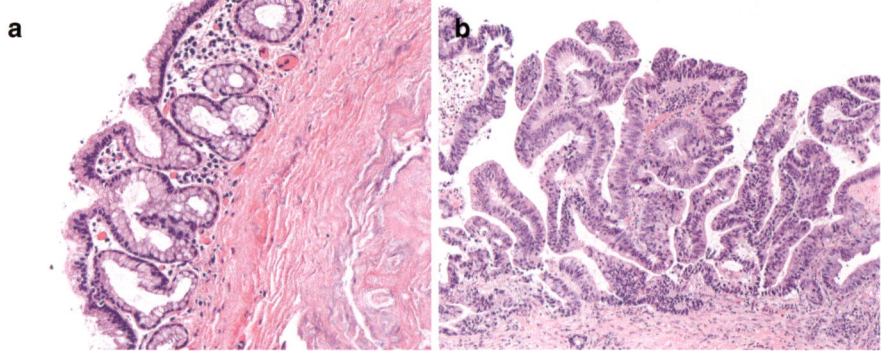

Fig. 3.6 (**a**) Low-grade dysplasia in IPMN characterized by regular, basal nuclei. (**b**) In high-grade dysplasia, the architecture is complex, and the cytology is pleomorphic (© 1998–2014 Mayo Foundation for Medical Education and Research. All rights reserved)

Such classification is important in prognosis and risk of associated invasive malignancy.

IPMNs must be sampled extensively, because approximately 30 % of them, most often main duct IPMN [21], are associated with an invasive component. The invasive component determines the prognosis, underscoring the need for a diligent search for foci of invasion. Microscopically, it can be challenging to distinguish invasion from intraductal spread of an IPMN into smaller branch ducts. The criteria for diagnosis of invasion include: perineural or angiolymphatic invasion, glands adjacent to muscular arteries or in peripancreatic fat, an infiltrative growth pattern, and variation in nuclear size of neoplastic cells with more than a 4:1 ratio between the largest and smallest tumor nuclei. Pools of mucin with floating neoplastic epithelial cells within the stroma are also diagnostic of invasion and must be distinguished from acellular extruded mucin.

While mutations in *KRAS*, *GNAS*, and *RNF43* have been identified which support the diagnosis of IPMN, mutations in these genes are also seen in MCN which renders detection of these genetic alterations as markers of neoplasia but not specific for either diagnosis [13, 14].

3.3   Serous Cystadenoma/Serous Cystic Neoplasm (SCN)

Pancreatic SCNs tend to occur in the body or tail of the pancreas; and as with MCN, females predominate with a female to male ratio of 3:1. SCN is a benign neoplasm and should be treated as such. These tumors are well circumscribed and have a spongelike cut surface due to the presence of multiple small cysts (Fig. 3.7). Although macrocystic/oligocystic examples occur, they are exceedingly rare [22]. In about 30 % of SCNs, there is a characteristic pathognomonic radiologic appearance imparted by calcification of a central stellate scar [23, 24].

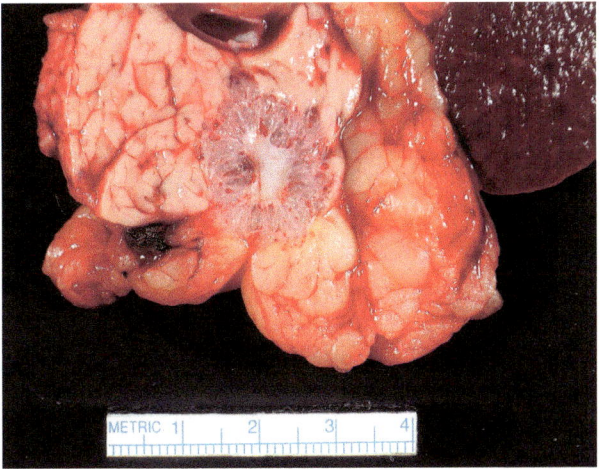

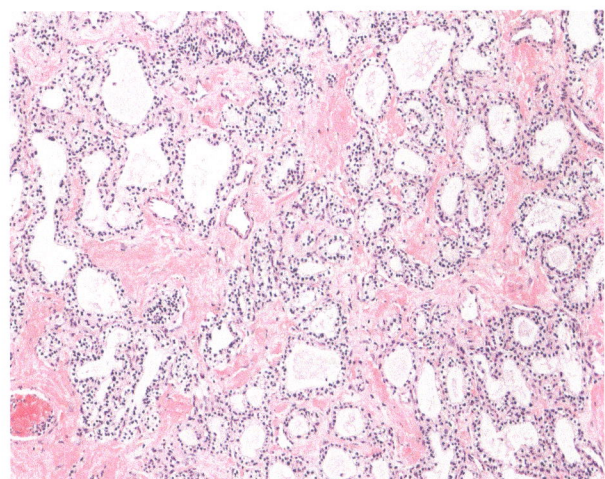

The microscopic appearance is also characteristic of SCN: a single layer of cuboidal cells with round, regular nuclei and a clear cytoplasm lining numerous small cystic spaces (Fig. 3.8). The cytoplasm of the cuboidal cells is clear due to glycogen, which can be confirmed by performing PAS stains with and without diastase digestion [25]. In rare instances, the epithelium can be attenuated focally, but other areas will show the expected microscopic findings. The sparse stroma between the cysts is mostly acellular, but islets of Langerhans and or pancreatic acini may be entrapped rarely in this stoma.

Macrocystic SCNs may be unilocular but are characteristically composed of larger and fewer cysts (measured in centimeters). The macrocystic SCN may not have a central stellate scar and may be less well circumscribed [26]. These variants should still be recognized readily on histopathologic exam because of the bland, clear, cuboidal epithelium lining the cysts. A solid variant of pancreatic SCN has

Fig. 3.9 The solid variant of
SCN. This variant needs to be
distinguished from clear cell
neuroendocrine neoplasm and
metastatic renal cell
carcinoma (© 1998–2014
Mayo Foundation for
Medical Education and
Research. All rights reserved)

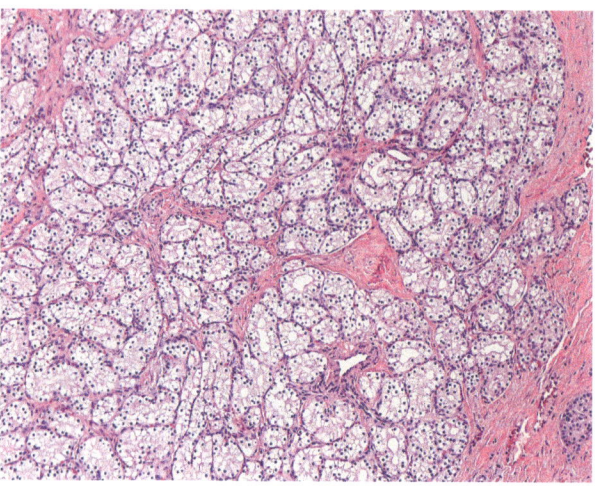

been described (Fig. 3.9) [27]. The neoplastic cells of this variant are arranged in
sheets or nests, a pattern that mimics the clear cell form of renal cell carcinoma or a
neuroendocrine carcinoma; renal cell carcinoma, however, shows more nuclear
atypia and expresses both vimentin and a wide-spectrum cytokeratin, while neuroendocrine carcinomas feature nuclei with a "salt and pepper" appearance to the chro-
matin and are strongly and diffusely positive for synaptophysin and chromogranin by
immunohistochemistry. In contrast, pancreatic SCNs are positive for cytokeratins,
MUC6, and inhibin, but SCNs do not express vimentin or the neuroendocrine marker
chromogranin [22]. Synaptophysin may be focally positive in pancreatic SCN [28].

Pancreatic SCNs are solitary; the presence of multiple tumors should raise consideration for von Hippel-Lindau syndrome [29]. This hereditary tumor predisposi-
tion syndrome also includes the association of serous cystic neoplasms with
neuroendocrine proliferation. The neuroendocrine component can be adjacent to or
intermingled with the serous cysts [29].

There are very rare examples of malignant pancreatic SCN (serous cystadenocarcinoma) [30]. Figure 3.10 shows a serous cystadenocarcinoma that recurred outside
the gastric wall. Note that the nuclei are larger and more variable than in usual serous
tumors, but there are no defined morphologic criteria for this diagnosis; malignancy
is defined by the presence of metastatic disease usually to the liver, regional lymph
nodes, or peritoneum [31]. These serous cystadenomas are quite rare, and their pos-
sibility does not support an aggressive approach to all patients with SCN.

3.4 Pancreatic Neuroendocrine Neoplasms with Cystic Change

Neuroendocrine neoplasms are usually solid but can undergo cystic degeneration
(Fig. 3.11). This degeneration creates a cystic appearance, but these are not true
cystic neoplasms, because they lack the defining characteristic of true cysts, that is,

Fig. 3.10 Serous cystadenocarcinoma recurrent as a mass in the gastric wall. While the nuclei are enlarged, the only reliable criterion for malignancy is metastatic/ recurrent disease (© 1998–2014 Mayo Foundation for Medical Education and Research. All rights reserved)

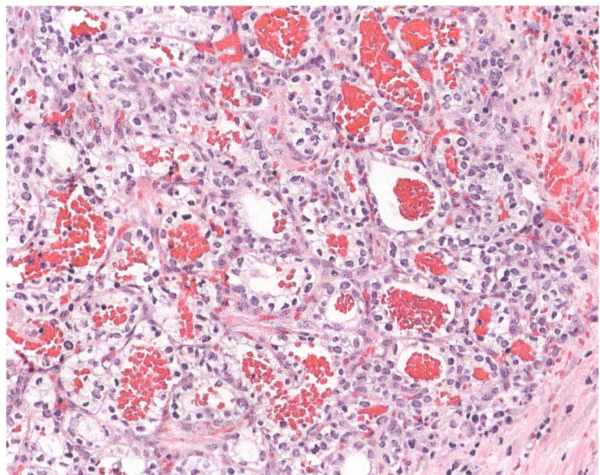

Fig. 3.11 Pancreatic neuroendocrine neoplasm with cystic degeneration. There is a small focus of solid pink tumor at 10 o'clock (© 1998–2014 Mayo Foundation for Medical Education and Research. All rights reserved)

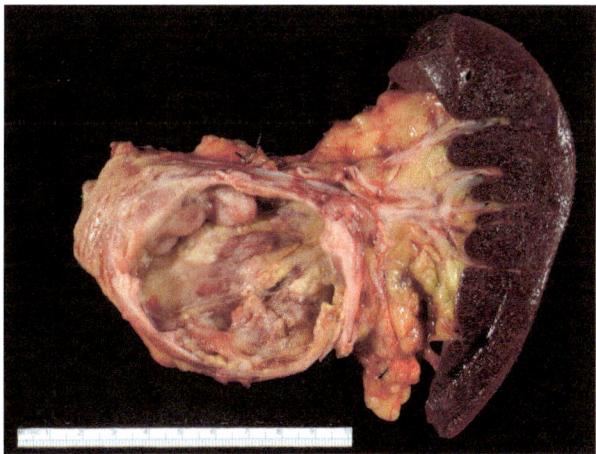

spaces lined by epithelium [32, 33]. Neuroendocrine carcinomas are often recognized easily because of their morphologic and immunohistochemical features. They are strongly and diffusely positive for synaptophysin and chromogranin and are negative for inhibin. The behavior of neuroendocrine neoplasms is determined by their stage and grade [34, 35].

3.5 Solid Pseudopapillary Neoplasm (SPN)

Solid pseudopapillary neoplasm has also been called Franz tumor, Hamoudi tumor, or solid and cystic neoplasm of the pancreas. These unique neoplasms have a marked female predilection (9:1) and usually affect young women (less than 35 years old) and even teenagers. SPN can arise in any part of the pancreas. SPN is not truly cystic

Fig. 3.12 SPN with the characteristic combination of fleshy, *red-brown* areas and hemorrhagic necrosis (© 1998–2014 Mayo Foundation for Medical Education and Research. All rights reserved)

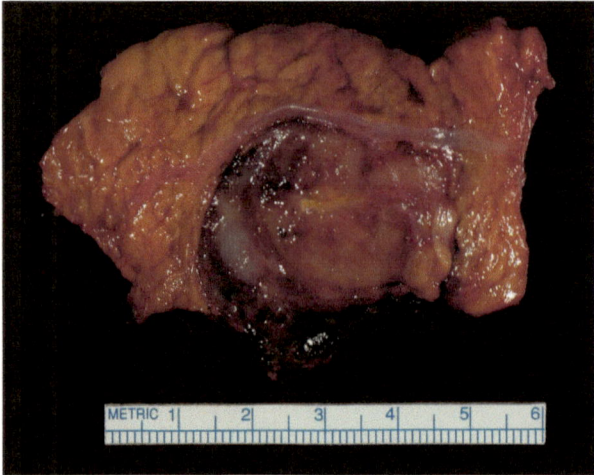

Fig. 3.13 The pseudopapillary appearance of SPN derives from the fact that tumor cells adjacent to vessels remain viable, while those away from vessels die and drop away (© 1998–2014 Mayo Foundation for Medical Education and Research. All rights reserved)

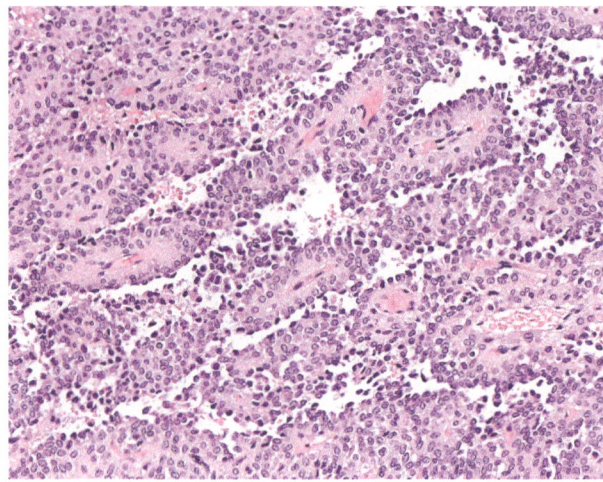

but commonly undergoes cystic degeneration to give the appearance of a solid and cystic mass [36]. The tumor is well circumscribed, but the appearance of the cut surface varies according to the degree of degenerative change, ranging from completely solid to almost completely hemorrhagic (Fig. 3.12). In the latter case, careful sampling at the periphery of the tumor may be necessary to make the correct diagnosis. The neoplasm is composed of monotonous cells with frequent nuclear grooves and cytoplasmic hyaline globules accompanied by a delicate capillary vasculature. Occasional clear cells can be seen. The neoplastic cells adjacent to the vasculature remain viable, while cells more remote from the blood vessels die, imparting a pseudopapillary and cystic appearance microscopically and macroscopically (Fig. 3.13). While grossly well circumscribed, these tumors are not encapsulated, and the border between tumor and pancreas can be irregular, but this finding is not a criterion for malignancy. Although SPN can mimic closely neuroendocrine neoplasms, SPN can be distinguished by careful review of the aforementioned microscopic features (nuclear grooves, hyaline globules, and pseudopapillary architecture) [37]. SPN also tend to have numerous foamy macrophages and cholesterol clefts, features not typical of neuroendocrine neoplasm. In difficult cases including needle biopsies, immunohistochemistry is invaluable in confirming the diagnosis. Strong nuclear expression of beta catenin is a very sensitive and specific diagnostic marker [38, 39]. SPN also express CD10, a progesterone receptor, and chymotrypsin [40]. Cytokeratin expression is either weak or absent [41]. Neuroendocrine markers are typically negative, but variable expression of synaptophysin or chromogranin can be seen [41]. Overall, the clinical course of SPN is benign with few cases of locally aggressive behavior, but metastases can occur [42, 43]; a very aggressive approach to these metastases even if they are distant is warranted [44].

3.6 Cystic Tumors with Acinar Lining

Most pancreatic acinar tumors are solid. There are very rare cystic neoplasms lined by acinar cells. Such neoplasms are usually benign (acinar cell cystadenoma), but there are vanishingly rare acinar cell cystadenocarcinomas. The cells lining the cysts are cuboidal and have zymogen granules. Their lineage can be confirmed immunohistochemically using an antibody to trypsin.

References

1. Thompson LD, et al. Mucinous cystic neoplasm (mucinous cystadenocarcinoma of low-grade malignant potential) of the pancreas: a clinicopathologic study of 130 cases. Am J Surg Pathol. 1999;23(1):1–16.
2. Zamboni G, et al. Mucinous cystic tumors of the pancreas: clinicopathological features, prognosis, and relationship to other mucinous cystic tumors. Am J Surg Pathol. 1999;23(4):410–22.
3. Masia R, et al. Pancreatic mucinous cystic neoplasm of the main pancreatic duct. Arch Pathol Lab Med. 2011;135(2):264–7.
4. Yamao K, et al. Clinicopathological features and prognosis of mucinous cystic neoplasm with ovarian-type stroma: a multi-institutional study of the Japan Pancreas Society. Pancreas. 2011;40(1):67–71.
5. Albores-Saavedra J, et al. Nonmucinous cystadenomas of the pancreas with pancreatobiliary phenotype and ovarian-like stroma. Am J Clin Pathol. 2013;139(5):599–604.
6. Baker ML, et al. Invasive mucinous cystic neoplasms of the pancreas. Exp Mol Pathol. 2012;93(3):345–9.
7. Lewis GH, et al. Prognosis of minimally invasive carcinoma arising in mucinous cystic neoplasms of the pancreas. Am J Surg Pathol. 2013;37(4):601–5.
8. Sarnaik AA, et al. Osteoclast-like giant cell tumor of the pancreas associated with a mucinous cystadenocarcinoma. Surgery. 2003;133(6):700–1.
9. van den Berg W, et al. Pancreatic mucinous cystic neoplasms with sarcomatous stroma: molecular evidence for monoclonal origin with subsequent divergence of the epithelial and sarcomatous components. Mod Pathol. 2000;13(1):86–91.

10. Adsay NV. Cystic neoplasia of the pancreas: pathology and biology. J Gastrointest Surg. 2008;12(3):401–4.
11. Volkan Adsay N. Cystic lesions of the pancreas. Mod Pathol. 2007;20 Suppl 1:S71–93.
12. Luttges J, et al. The mucin profile of noninvasive and invasive mucinous cystic neoplasms of the pancreas. Am J Surg Pathol. 2002;26(4):466–71.
13. Furukawa T, et al. Whole-exome sequencing uncovers frequent GNAS mutations in intraductal papillary mucinous neoplasms of the pancreas. Sci Rep. 2011;1:161.
14. Wu J, et al. Whole-exome sequencing of neoplastic cysts of the pancreas reveals recurrent mutations in components of ubiquitin-dependent pathways. Proc Natl Acad Sci U S A. 2011;108(52):21188–93.
15. Tanaka M, et al. International consensus guidelines for management of intraductal papillary mucinous neoplasms and mucinous cystic neoplasms of the pancreas. Pancreatol. 2006;6(1–2):17–32.
16. Crippa S, et al. Mucin-producing neoplasms of the pancreas: an analysis of distinguishing clinical and epidemiologic characteristics. ClinClin Gastroenterol Hepatol. 2010;8(2):213–9.
17. Nara S, et al. Preoperative evaluation of invasive and noninvasive intraductal papillary-mucinous neoplasms of the pancreas: clinical, radiological, and pathological analysis of 123 cases. Pancreas. 2009;38(1):8–16.
18. Schnelldorfer T, et al. Experience with 208 resections for intraductal papillary mucinous neoplasm of the pancreas. Arch Surg. 2008;143(7):639–46; discussion 646.
19. Matthaei H, et al. Cystic precursors to invasive pancreatic cancer. Nature reviews. Gastroenterol Hepatol. 2011;8(3):141–50.
20. Adsay NV, et al. Pathologically and biologically distinct types of epithelium in intraductal papillary mucinous neoplasms: delineation of an "intestinal" pathway of carcinogenesis in the pancreas. Am J Surg Pathol. 2004;28(7):839–48.
21. Schmidt CM, et al. Intraductal papillary mucinous neoplasms: predictors of malignant and invasive pathology. Ann Surg. 2007;246(4):644–51; discussion 651–4.
22. Kosmahl M, et al. Serous cystic neoplasms of the pancreas: an immunohistochemical analysis revealing alpha-inhibin, neuron-specific enolase, and MUC6 as new markers. Am J Surg Pathol. 2004;28(3):339–46.
23. Friedman AC, Lichtenstein JE, Dachman AH. Cystic neoplasms of the pancreas. Radiological-pathological correlation. Radiology. 1983;149(1):45–50.
24. Zaheer A, et al. Incidentally detected cystic lesions of the pancreas on CT: review of literature and management suggestions. Abdom Imaging. 2013;38(2):331–41.
25. Bogomoletz WV, et al. Cystadenoma of the pancreas: a histological, histochemical and ultrastructural study of seven cases. Histopathology. 1980;4(3):309–20.
26. Egawa N, et al. Serous oligocystic and ill-demarcated adenoma of the pancreas: a variant of serous cystic adenoma. Virchows Archiv. 1994;424(1):13–7.
27. Perez-Ordonez B, et al. Solid serous adenoma of the pancreas. The solid variant of serous cystadenoma? Am J Surg Pathol. 1996;20(11):1401–5.
28. Kanehira K, Khoury T. Neuroendocrine markers expression in pancreatic serous cystadenoma. Appl immunohistochem Mol morphol. 2011;19(2):141–6.
29. Hammel PR, et al. Pancreatic involvement in von Hippel-Lindau disease. The Groupe Francophone d'Etude de la Maladie de von Hippel-Lindau. Gastroenterology. 2000;119(4):1087–95.
30. Bramis K, et al. Serous cystadenocarcinoma of the pancreas: report of a case and management reflections. World J Surg Oncol. 2012;10:51.
31. Matsumoto T, et al. Malignant serous cystic neoplasm of the pancreas: report of a case and review of the literature. J Clin Gastroenterol. 2005;39(3):253–6.
32. Singhi AD, et al. Cystic pancreatic neuroendocrine tumors: a clinicopathologic study. Am J Surg Pathol. 2012;36(11):1666–73.
33. Bordeianou L, et al. Cystic pancreatic endocrine neoplasms: a distinct tumor type? J Am Coll Surg. 2008;206(3):1154–8.

34. Qadan M, et al. Reassessment of the Current American Joint Committee on Cancer Staging System for Pancreatic Neuroendocrine Tumors. J Am Coll Surg. 2014;218:188–195.
35. Ito H, et al. Surgery and staging of pancreatic neuroendocrine tumors: a 14-year experience. J Gastrointest Surg. 2010;14(5):891–8.
36. Kosmahl M, et al. Solid-pseudopapillary tumor of the pancreas: its origin revisited. Virchows Archiv. 2000;436(5):473–80.
37. Meriden Z, et al. Hyaline globules in neuroendocrine and solid-pseudopapillary neoplasms of the pancreas: a clue to the diagnosis. Am J Surg Pathol. 2011;35(7):981–8.
38. Tanaka Y, et al. Usefulness of beta-catenin immunostaining for the differential diagnosis of solid-pseudopapillary neoplasm of the pancreas. Am J Surg Pathol. 2002;26(6):818–20.
39. Abraham SC, et al. Solid-pseudopapillary tumors of the pancreas are genetically distinct from pancreatic ductal adenocarcinomas and almost always harbor beta-catenin mutations. Am J Pathol. 2002;160(4):1361–9.
40. Notohara K, et al. Solid-pseudopapillary tumor of the pancreas: immunohistochemical localization of neuroendocrine markers and CD10. Am J Surg Pathol. 2000;24(10):1361–71.
41. Kim MJ, Jang SJ, Yu E. Loss of E-cadherin and cytoplasmic-nuclear expression of beta-catenin are the most useful immunoprofiles in the diagnosis of solid-pseudopapillary neoplasm of the pancreas. Hum Pathol. 2008;39(2):251–8.
42. Yang F, et al. Solid pseudopapillary tumor of the pancreas: a case series of 26 consecutive patients. Am J Surg. 2009;198(2):210–5.
43. Wang XG, et al. Clinicopathologic features and surgical outcome of solid pseudopapillary tumor of the pancreas: analysis of 17 cases. World J Surg Oncol. 2013;11:38.
44. Tipton SG, Smyrk TC, Sarr MG. Malignant potential of solid pseudopapillary neoplasm of the pancreas. Br J Surg. 2006;93:733–7.

Clinical Features and Laboratory Investigation

George H. Sakorafas, Vassileios Smyrniotis, and Michael G. Sarr

4.1 Clinical Presentation

PCNs are often asymptomatic and diagnosed incidentally, usually on cross-sectional imaging during the workup of patients for vague and unrelated abdominal complains [1]. In patients who present with symptoms, the complains are often nonspecific, such as nausea, vomiting, abdominal or back pain, jaundice, pancreatitis, steatorrhea, weight loss, fatigue, malaise, fullness/palpable mass, etc. [1–4]. Clinical symptomatology (in particular jaundice, substantial weight loss, and pain) is associated with a high risk of malignancy [5].

In SCNs, clinical symptomatology is observed more commonly in the large (>4 cm) compared to smaller (<4 cm) SCNs (72 % vs. 22 %, $p < 0.001$) [6]. Most symptoms appear to be related to a mass effect (pressure rather than infiltration). Systemic symptoms, such as fatigue, malaise, weight loss, etc. (indicating malignant disease), are extremely rare.

In contrast to SCNs, MCNs are more commonly symptomatic, probably because of their larger size and their more aggressive, local biologic behavior. In patients with MCNs, the presence of clinical symptomatology (especially back pain, jaundice, or systemic manifestations) should increase the suspicion for underlying malignancy [4].

G.H. Sakorafas, MD (✉)
Department of Surgical Oncology, Saint Savvas Cancer Hospital,
Arkadias 19-21, Athens 11526, Greece
e-mail: georgesakorafas@yahoo.com

V. Smyrniotis, MD
4th Department of Surgery, Attikon University Hospital, Chanioti 22, Athens 15452, Greece
e-mail: vsmyrniotis@hotmail.com

M.G. Sarr, MD
Department of Surgery, Mayo Clinic, 200 First Street SW, Rochester, MN 55905, USA
e-mail: sarr.michael@mayo.edu

© Springer-Verlag Italia 2015
G.H. Sakorafas et al. (eds.), *Pancreatic Cystic Neoplasms:*
From Imaging to Differential Diagnosis and Management,
DOI 10.1007/978-88-470-5708-1_4

As in SCN and MCN, most IPMNs are diagnosed incidentally, and patients are often asymptomatic. Symptomatic patients with IPMN (mainly the main-duct variant) may present with abdominal pain, jaundice, new onset of diabetes, and pale stools. Recurrent episodes of pancreatitis, "idiopathic" chronic pancreatitis, or rarely acute cholangitis are other possible clinical scenarios caused by the obstruction of the ductal system from mucus or papillary projections within the duct [7]. In the past, these patients were misdiagnosed and treated as suffering from idiopathic large duct chronic pancreatitis. The clinical presentation typical of pancreatic ductal adenocarcinoma (i.e., painless jaundice, weight loss, new onset diabetes, etc.) may be observed in some malignant main-duct IPMNs [8–10]. In contrast, branch-duct IPMNs are most often asymptomatic compared to main-duct IPMN, especially when the lesion is <3 cm. IPMNs have also been associated with other syndromes, such as Peutz-Jeghers syndrome, familial adenomatous polyposis (FAP), and their clinical manifestations [11, 12]. IPMN also has a very interesting but still unexplained increased association with typical ductal adenocarcinoma of the pancreas. In addition, several authors have shown that 30 % of IPMN patients have a history of extrapancreatic neoplasms, particularly in the stomach, colon, or rectum [13, 14].

Other rare PCNs are typically diagnosed incidentally on imaging studies in individuals without specific symptoms. Solid pseudopapillary neoplasms (SPNs) are commonly asymptomatic [15–18]; however, the larger lesions may by symptomatic. When present, clinical symptoms are often vague and may include abdominal bloating and distention, discomfort, pain, presence of a palpable mass, anorexia, nausea, weight loss, etc. [19–21]. Rare cases of pancreatitis, biliary obstruction, and intra-abdominal bleeding due to tumor rupture have also been reported [19–23]. Although SPNs often have an indolent course, they are malignant lesions; if left untreated, SPNs may invade into adjacent organs and major vessels [24]; these cases are typically associated with clinical symptomatology. Most cystic pancreatic neuroendocrine tumors (PNETs) are nonfunctioning and are discovered on abdominal imaging [25–28]. In about 25 % of patients, cystic PNETs are associated with a MEN syndrome [29]. Other rare PCNs are either asymptomatic or associated with nonspecific, clinical manifestations.

4.2   FNA Analysis of the Cystic Fluid

Because imaging alone has limitations regarding definitive diagnosis, fine-needle aspiration (FNA) and examination of the cystic fluid (cytology/biochemical analysis) have been studied extensively and have demonstrated clinical utility (Table 4.1). FNA is performed under image guidance, most commonly endoscopically (endoscopic ultrasound [EUS]-guided), but occasionally percutaneously (CT- or US-guided). EUS is preferred for image guidance, because with the tumor being closer to the transducer, the imaging resolution is greater. Moreover, by a transgastric or transduodenal aspiration, the endoscopic approach has fewer potential complications.

Table 4.1 Analysis of cyst fluid aspirate

	Pseudocyst	SCN	MCN	IPMN	SPPT	Lymphoepithelial cyst
Cytologic findings	"Dirty" material, macrophages, and other inflammatory cells	Negative, or cellular sheets of glycogen-containing, cuboidal cells	Mucin-containing columnar cells; small papillary sheets	Papillary clusters lined by mucin-containing columnar cells; atypia	Branching papillae, cuboidal or cylindrical cells, high cellularity, myxoid stroma	Squamous cells, keratin debris with or without lymphocytes, and cholesterol crystals
Laboratory analyses						
Viscosity	Low	Low	High	High	NA	Low
Mucin	None	None	Present	Present	NA	None
CEA level (ng/ml)[a]	Low, usually <5	Low, usually <5	High, >5	High, >5	NA	Low, <5
Amylase activity	High (>250 U/l)	Low (<250 U/l)	Low (<250 U/l)	Low to medium (<250 U/l)[b]	Low	Low

Modified from Sakorafas et al. [48]

NA not applicable (cyst aspiration is rarely performed during the diagnostic work-up)

[a]CEA <5 ng/ml excludes a mucinous neoplasm. CEA >192 ng/ml used to differentiate SCN from MCN and IPMN

[b]Amylase activity increased in IPMNs

4.2.1 Image-Guided FNA Cytology

Cytology may be helpful for differentiating mucinous from non-mucinous cysts through identifying mucin-producing cells (Table 4.1). When positive, the characteristic cytology of SCNs is that of cellular sheets of low-cuboidal, glycogen-containing cells without cellular atypia. The cytoplasm is clear and without vacuoles and intracellular cytoplasmic inclusions. SCNs demonstrate positive immunostaining for cytokeratins AE_1 and AE_3 and positive staining with the periodic acid-Schiff reaction (Fig. 4.1) [30–33].

In contrast, low-grade MCNs are characterized by honeycomb sheets and clusters of columnar, mucin-containing cells with rare, small, papillary sheets [34, 35]. In addition, MCNs have abundant mucin in their background, which differentiates MCNs from SCNs [35]. Because of the extreme heterogeneity of the epithelial lining of MCNs, one must remember that there may be marked discrepancies between the cytologic typing and the subsequent histologic diagnosis of these neoplasms. Importantly, however, the degree of cytologic atypia has been shown to be predictive of malignancy [36]. Also cytology may diagnose malignant cystic lesions (e.g., cystadenocarcinoma) by demonstrating malignant cells or cells with high-grade atypia (dysplasia) in the aspirated cystic fluid [37].

IPMNs are characterized on FNA cytology by the presence of papillary clusters lined by columnar, mucin-containing cells, usually with some degree of atypia [38]. Although low-grade MCNs may have a few papillary clusters, the papillary projections in MCNs are usually not as tall, abundant, and striking as the clusters observed in IPMNs. One study suggested the presence of hemosiderin-laden macrophages in the aspirated fluid as a finding supporting the diagnosis of SCN [39]. In this study, hemosiderin-laden macrophages were identified in 11 of the 21 cases of SCNs (52 %) but in only 2 % of IPMNs and MCNs and in only 9 % of pseudocysts (Fig. 4.1e); at the current time, however, the presence of hemosiderin-laden macrophages is not considered a reliable diagnostic feature of SCN and can only serve as a surrogate marker to suggest the diagnosis of SCN. In contrast to PCNs, FNA of pancreatic pseudocysts yields a "dirty" material with macrophages and other inflammatory cells, proteinaceous precipitates, and calcified debris.

4.2.2 Analysis of Aspirated Cystic Fluid

Macroscopically, the aspirated fluid of SCNs is typically thin, clear, and without mucin, but on occasion may be bloody [40] (Table 4.1). In contrast, the aspirated fluid in mucinous neoplasms is thick, viscid, and of a mucinous nature; the mucinous nature of the fluid can often be appreciated grossly in the endoscopy suite when smears are made. A typical analysis of the aspirated cystic fluid would include biochemical testing (for mucin, tumor markers, and amylase) and potentially for molecular analysis.

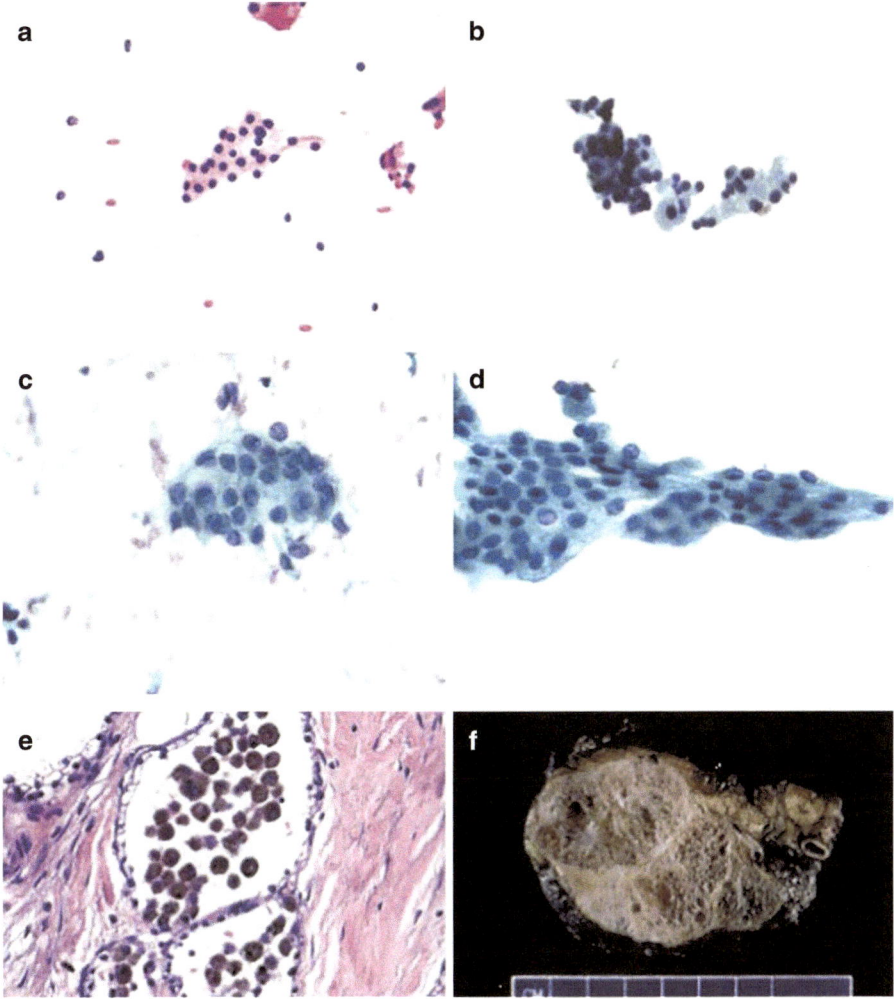

Fig. 4.1 (**a**) Direct smear of a resected SCN. Cuboidal cells with small round nuclei and clear cytoplasm (H & E). (**b**) FNA. Cluster of bland, cuboidal to columnar epithelial cells with ampho-philic cytoplasm and round nuclei. (**c**) FNA. A cluster of bland, cuboidal to columnar epithelial cells with clear cytoplasm and round nuclei, consistent with serous epithelial lining (Papanicolaou stain).(**d**) FNA. A sheet of bland epithelial cells with round to oval nuclei and atypical cytoplasm, oriented in a streaming fashion and consistent with gastrointestinal epithelial contamination (Papanicolaou stain). (**e**) Hemosiderin-laden macrophages within a cystic lumen of a serous cyst-adenoma (H& E). (**f**) Macroscopic photograph of a pancreatic resection revealing a multiloculated, cystic lesion with central fibrous tissue (With permission from Belsley et al. [30])

Mucin

A positive mucin stain or a high viscosity (indicative of mucin) is highly specific for the premalignant or overly malignant mucinous neoplasms (i.e., MCN and IPMN) and can be used for their differential diagnosis from SCN and usually from pseudocysts as well [41]. Unfortunately, easily used and reliable assays for mucin are not readily available; some groups no longer utilize mucin stains because of their difficulty in preparation.

CEA

The CEA level of the cyst fluid is the most accurate test for determining the cyst to be mucinous and for differentiating a mucinous neoplasm from a SCN with a reasonable reliability [42]. Interestingly, in the study by Brugge et al., no combination of tests, including appearance on EUS, was more accurate than CEA alone [43]. The best cutoff level for CEA may vary from lab to lab, depending on the assay used, but many centers, particularly in the USA, use a CEA level of 192 ng/ml as diagnostically sensitive (75 %) and specific (84 %) for differentiating mucinous from non-mucinous neoplasms (overall diagnostic accuracy 79 % for mucinous lesions) [43]. A CEA level of <5 ng/ml is equally sensitive for excluding a mucinous neoplasm and has a 50 % sensitivity and 95 % specificity for the identification of SCA or pseudocyst [40, 44, 45] (Table 4.1). Cyst CEA levels are not, however, a reliable marker to differentiate benign from any of the malignant mucinous cystic neoplasms [46]. Also, CEA cannot differentiate mucinous cystadenoma from IPMN, because CEA levels are increased in all mucinous cysts [47].

Amylase

Amylase activity in the cystic fluid is of limited diagnostic value, except that a high amylase activity (>5 times the serum activity) suggests that there is a communication between the cyst and the pancreatic ductal system, thereby excluding SCNs and MCNs (Table 4.1) [48]. High amylase activities do not always help in differentiating IPMN from pancreatic pseudocysts, because both entities communicate directly with the pancreatic ductal system, but very high amylase levels (>10,000 U/l) are associated with 98 % specificity for a pseudocyst in the appropriate setting. Amylase activities in the cyst fluid of less than 250 U/l virtually excludes pseudocyst [44]. High levels of cyst fluid amylase (and/or lipase) are also seen in patients with all forms of IPMN, because the cyst has communication with the pancreatic duct (Table 4.1).

Other Tumor Markers

CA 19-9, CA 72-4, CA 125, and CA 15.3 may be present in greater concentrations in MCNs, but their diagnostic value is limited, and their use for making therapeutic decisions is not recommended in clinical practice.

Genetic Markers

More recently, analysis of the intracystic fluid for telomerase activity, DNA quality, and a panel of mutations has proved promising though not yet fully accepted in differentiation of benign versus malignant lesions [49]. Only a few drops of fluid are required; thus, this molecular analysis can be applied to most cyst aspirates. Measurement of allelic loss amplitude has a sensitivity of 67 % and specificity of 66 % for mucinous cystic lesions [15, 50]. The presence of a k-*ras* mutation is highly specific (96 %) for mucinous lesions but has a low sensitivity of 45 % [50, 51]. Chai et al. assessed the performance of CEA, cytology, and k-*ras* mutations in the cyst fluid for diagnosing mucinous cysts. They found an increased cyst fluid CEA or abnormal cytology to be the most sensitive test to diagnose mucinous cysts; however, k-*ras* mutation identified mucinous cysts in only 2 of 25 (8 %) patients in whom CEA and cytology were non-diagnostic [52]. Negative k-*ras* testing does not exclude a mucinous cyst; however, a positive k-*ras* mutation supports strongly the diagnosis of a mucinous cyst even when cyst fluid CEA is not increased [53]. It should also be noted that K-*ras* mutations can also be present in normal and inflammatory pancreatic ducts [54]. The value of this expensive test to predict the risk of progression to malignancy requires further confirmation in prospective trials.

4.2.3   Comments

EUS-guided transluminal FNA is a well-tolerated and safe procedure when performed by an experienced operator. EUS, however, remains a specialized examination limited to a few centers with the necessary equipment and especially within the obligate experience of the endoscopist. Analysis of the cystic fluid depends on the ability of local cytologic and laboratory testing and is not available routinely. Potential complications of needle aspirations of cystic fluid include bleeding due to vascular injury (clinically relevant bleeding, <1 %; self-limiting intracystic hemorrhage ~6 %), pancreatitis (~1–3 %), infection (<1 %), and, at least in theory, the seeding of malignant cells along the tract of the needle [36, 55, 56]. Periprocedural antibiotics are used commonly to decrease the risk of introduced intracystic infection. Most endoscopists also tend to remove as much fluid as possible to decrease the theoretic risk of bacterial inoculation of the fluid.

Consideration should be given to the size of the lesion and the size of the individual "cysts," because aspirates may be very limited for small lesions which might preclude or complicate cyst analysis and cytology. A small (<1 ml) volume of the aspirates may be due to the high viscosity of the aspirated fluid (due to the presence of mucin) in MCNs or to the small size of the cysts in the cystic lesion of SCNs [57]. Moreover, the size of the cystic lesion is of clinical importance when deciding about the indication to perform EUS-guided FNA. There is no uniform agreement in relation to the cutoff size for EUS-guided aspiration. Some investigators have proposed a cutoff diameter of 1.5 cm [58, 59]; these groups rarely perform EUS-guided FNA in smaller lesions. A size of >1.5 cm was chosen based on the likelihood that it would allow the aspiration of an adequate volume of fluid for analysis [59]. Others use a threshold of 2.0 cm [60, 61], while some groups do not quote specific size criteria [62, 63]. A few centers advocate EUS in all patients with asymptomatic cysts [64, 65].

Some reports are very enthusiastic about the value of the combination of EUS and FNA in predicting which lesions require resection, with reported sensitivities and specificity of 97 and 100 %, respectively [34]; in contrast, other studies report less convincing results. In a large, prospective, multicenter trial, cyst fluid cytology had a high specificity (83 %) but a low sensitivity (35 %) for distinguishing mucinous vs. non-mucinous cysts [43]. In this study, the sensitivity for diagnosing malignancy was only 22 % [43]. Others have reported diagnostic accuracy of EUS-guided FNA ranging only between 10 and 60 % [31, 33, 66]. Genevay et al. re-reviewed the cytology slides of 112 patients with histologically confirmed, mucinous cysts of the pancreas. They found that high-grade atypia (dysplasia) in the epithelial cells had a specificity of 85 % and sensitivity of 72 % for predicting malignancy in mucinous cysts [37]. Pais et al. reported that EUS-guided FNA cytology proved helpful with a sensitivity, specificity, and accuracy for the diagnosis of malignancy of 75, 91, and 86 % respectively [46]. The reported variations in diagnostic accuracy likely are due to differences in the sampling technique, the experience of the endoscopist or cytopathologist, and the thoroughness with which clinicopathologic correlation was accomplished.

The low cellularity of the aspirated pancreatic cyst fluid is a major limitation of FNA cytology for the differentiation between the different types of PCNs. As a result, cytologic examination of the cyst fluid is often non-diagnostic. In the study by Huang et al. [31], 32 % of the 28 cases were classified initially as "non-diagnostic specimens" or as having "no malignant cells." Even in re-aspirated specimens, the interpretations were usually unchanged. In contrast, when such samples are positive, the specificity is high [31, 67]. As reported by Al-Haddad et al. [68], brushing the cyst wall during FNA increases the diagnostic yield of EUS-guided FNA; in their study of 37 patients with a pancreatic cystic lesion, the sensitivity of cyst fluid FNA for detecting intracellular mucin was 23 % but increased to 62 % by brushing the cyst wall [68].

The accuracy of preoperative differential diagnosis can also be increased by obtaining image-guided "mini-biopsies" (Tru-Cut or core tissue biopsies) from the solid component of a cystic neoplasm or from the wall of the cyst (cyst wall puncture) [69, 70]. Recently, although the technology to allow an endoscopic, Tru-Cut core tissue biopsy has been developed, it is not yet available widely. Early data with EUS-guided Tru-Cut biopsies of PCNs have shown very promising results. In the study by Levy et al., 5 of 6 SCNs were identified correctly on a Tru-Cut biopsy [71]. In the study by Belsley et al. [30], both biopsies performed with the Tru-Cut technique were diagnostic, without any procedural complications reported.

Apart from the sampling error, "contamination" of the aspirates from the normal (mucus-producing) epithelium of the gastrointestinal tract during the passage of the needle may pose another problem in interpreting the results of EUS-guided, FNA cytology (Fig. 4.1d). Such an error may result in the misdiagnosis of a SCN as a mucinous neoplasm. Indeed, caution should be taken not to misinterpret mucin or mucin-producing cells as the mucinous material or epithelial cells of a MCN [72]. Mucin from the gastrointestinal tract tends to be thinner, wispier, and devoid of degenerated epithelial cells and the inflammation more typical of MCN [67, 72]. Unfortunately, this distinction is not always easy, because the features can overlap. Cell block material and ancillary tests (i.e., stains for glucagon, cystic levels of carcinoembryonic antigen (CEA), amylase activity, viscosity, etc.) may help to clarify the differential diagnosis, but only if the results are truly informative. Moreover, epithelial cells from the GI tract tend to form large, cohesive, monolayered sheets consisting of uniform, columnar cells without cytologic atypia and often with a luminal edge. These columnar cells usually do not contain abundant cytoplasmic mucin, and thus the cell border is not as prominent as that in MCN cells. Incarcerated, mucin-producing goblet cells are a constant feature of incidentally sampled duodenal epithelium; also, the openings of the crypts of Lieberkuhn or the pits may be seen in some cell groups [31, 67, 72]. In contrast, MCN cells are characterized by a mucin-rich columnar epithelium with thick mucin in the background. Although MCN cells may appear extremely bland, they often exhibit at least focally some cytologic atypia and architectural complexity [72].

From a practical point of view, it should be emphasized that when the imaging features of the cystic lesion are virtually diagnostic, FNA can be omitted, and the lesion should then be managed appropriately (see below). FNA should also be omitted when the cystic lesion is symptomatic, because in this case, resection is clearly indicated. FNA should probably be entertained only when its results may change the therapeutic plan, e.g., when high-quality, cross-sectional imaging reveals nondiagnostic findings or when the clinical and morphologic characters of the cystic lesion have changed during follow-up [73]. Another potential indication of FNA is when a non-operative approach is considered for a presumed SCN not diagnosed confidentially on cross-sectional imaging. In this case, if the results of FNA analysis of the cystic fluid are compatible with a MCN, the conservative approach should be reevaluated.

References

1. Valsangkar N, Morales-Oyarvide V, Thayer S, Ferrone C, Wargo J, Warshaw A, et al. 851 resected cystic tumors of the pancreas: a 33-year experience at the Massachusetts general hospital. Surgery. 2012;152(3 Suppl 1):S4–12.
2. Reddy RP, Smyrk TC, Zapiach M, Levy MJ, Pearson RK, Clain JE, et al. Pancreatic mucinous cystic neoplasm defined by ovarian stroma: demographics, clinical features, and prevalence of cancer. Clin Gastroenterol Hepatol. 2004;2:1026–31.
3. Kimura W, Moriya T, Hanada K, Abe H, Yanagisawa A, Fukushima N, Ohike N, Shimizu M, Hatori T, Fujita N, et al. Multicenter study of SCN of the Japan pancreas society: a multi-institutional study of 172 patients. Pancreas. 2012;41:380–7.
4. Crippa S, Salvia R, Warshaw AL, Dominguez I, Bassi C, Falconi M, et al. Mucinous cystic neoplasm of the pancreas is not an aggressive entity: lessons from 163 resected patients. Ann Surg. 2008;247(4):571–9.
5. Lennon AM, Wolfgang C. Cystic neoplasms of the pancreas. J Gastrointest Surg. 2013;17:645–53.
6. Tseng JF, Warshaw AL, Sahani DV, Lauwers GY, Rattner DW, Fernandez-del Castillo C. Serous cystadenoma of the pancreas: tumor growth rates and recommendations for treatment. Ann Surg. 2005;242:413–9.
7. Tibayan F, Vierra M, Mindelzun B, Tsang D, McClenathan J, Young H, Trueblood HW. Clinical presentation of mucin-secreting tumors of the pancreas. Am J Surg. 2000;179:349–51.
8. Sohn TA, Yeo CJ, Cameron JL, Hruban RH, Fukushima N, Campbell KA, Lillemoe KD. Intraductal papillary mucinous neoplasms of the pancreas: an updated experience. Ann Surg. 2004;239:788–97.

9. D'Angelica M, Brennan MF, Suriawinata AA, Klimstra D, Conlon KC. Intraductal papillary mucinous neoplasms of the pancreas: an analysis of clinicopathologic features and outcome. Ann Surg. 2004;239:400–8.

10. Salvia R, Fernández-del Castillo C, Bassi C, Thayer SP, Falconi M, Mantovani W, et al. Main-duct intraductal papillary mucinous neoplasms of the pancreas: clinical predictors of malignancy and long-term survival following resection. Ann Surg. 2004;239:678–87.

11. Maire F, Hammel P, Terris B, Olschwang S, O'Toole D, Sauvanet A, Palazzo L, Ponsot P, Laplane B, Levy P, et al. Intraductal papillary and mucinous pancreatic tumour: a new extra-colonic tumour in familial adenomatous polyposis. Gut. 2002;51:446–9.

12. Sato N, Rosty C, Jansen M, Fukushima N, Ueki T, Yeo CJ, Cameron JL, Iacobuzio-Donahue CA, Hruban RH, Goggins M. STK11/LKB1 Peutz-Jeghers gene inactivation in intraductal papillary-mucinous neoplasms of the pancreas. Am J Pathol. 2001;159:2017–22.

13. Sugiyama M, Atomi Y. Extrapancreatic neoplasms occur with unusual frequency in patients with intraductal papillary mucinous tumors of the pancreas. Am J Gastroenterol. 1999;94:470–3.

14. Adsay NV. Intraductal papillary mucinous neoplasms of the pancreas: pathology and molecular genetics. J Gastrointest Surg. 2002;6:656–9.

15. Mohamadnejad M, Eloubeidi MA. Cystic lesions of the pancreas. Arch Iran Med. 2013;16:233–9.

16. Klimstra DS, Wenig BM, Heffess CS. Solid-pseudopapillary tumor of the pancreas: a typically cystic carcinoma of low malignant potential. Semin Diagn Pathol. 2000;17:66–81.

17. Buetow PC, Buck JL, Pantongrag-Brown L, et al. Solid and papillary epithelial neoplasm of the pancreas: imaging-pathologic correlation on 56 cases. Radiology. 1996;199:707–11.

18. Coleman KL, Doherty MC, Bigler SA. Solid-pesudopapillary tumor of the pancreas. Radiographics. 2003;6:1644–8.

19. Papavramidis T, Papavramidis S. Solid pseudopapillary tumors of the pancreas: review of 718 patients reported in english literature. J Am Coll Surg. 2005;200:965–72.

20. Tipton SG, Smyrk TC, Sarr MG, Thompson GB. Malignant potential of solid pseudopapillary neoplasm of the pancreas. Br J Surg. 2006;93:733–7.

21. Roggin KK, Chennat J, Oto A, et al. Pancreatic cystic neoplasm. Curr Probl Surg. 2010;47:459–510.

22. Casadei R, Santini D, Calculli L, et al. Pancreatic solid-cystic papillary tumor: clinical features, imaging findings and operative management. JOP. 2006;7:137–44.

23. Mao C, Guvendi M, Domenico DR, et al. Papillary cystic and solid tumors of the pancreas: a pancreatic embryonic tumor? Study of three cases and cumulative review of the world's literature. Surgery. 1995;118:821–8.

24. Santini D, Poli F, Lega S. Solid-papillary tumors of the pancreas: histopathology. JOP. 2006;7:131–6.

25. Ligneau B, Lombard-Bohas C, Partensky C, et al. Cystic endocrine tumors of the pancreas: clinical, radiologic, and histopathologic features in 13 cases. Am J Surg Pathol. 2001;25:752–60.

26. Buetow PC, Parrino TV, Buck JL, et al. Islet cell tumors of the pancreas: pathologic-imaging correlation among size, necroses and cysts, calcification, malignant behavior, and function status. AJR Am J Roentgenol. 1995;165:1175–9.

27. Ahrendt SA, Komorowski RA, Demeure MJ, Wilson SD, Pitt HA. Cystic pancreatic neuroendocrine tumors: is preoperative diagnosis possible? J Gastrointest Surg. 2002;6:66–74.

28. Goh BK, Ooi LL, Tan YM, Cheow PC, Chung YF, Chow PK, et al. Clinico-pathologic features of cystic pancreatic endocrine neoplasms and a comparison with their solid counterparts. Eur J Surg Oncol. 2006;32:553–6.

29. Federle MP, McGrath KM. Cystic neoplasms of the pancreas. Gastroenterol Clin North Am. 2007;36:365–76.

30. Belsley NA, Pitman MB, Lauwers GY, Brugge WR, Deshpande V. Serous cystadenoma of the pancreas. Cancer (Cancer Cytopathol). 2008;114:102–10.

31. Huang P, Staerkel G, Sneige N, Gong Y. Fine-needle aspiration of pancreatic serous cystadenoma. Cytologic features and diagnostic pitfalls. Cancer Cytopathol. 2006;108:239–49.
32. Lal A, Bourtsos EP, DeFrias DV, Nemcek AA, Nayar R. Microcystic adenoma of the pancreas: clinical, radiologic, and cytologic features. Cancer. 2004;102:288–94.
33. Nguyen GK, Suen KC, Villanueva RR. Needle aspiration cytology of pancreatic cystic lesions. Diagn Cytopathol. 1997;17:177–82.
34. Frossard JL, Amouyal P, Amouyal G, Palazzo L, Amaris J, Soldan M, et al. Performance of endoscopically-guided fine needle aspiration and biopsy in the diagnosis of pancreatic cystic lesions. Am J Gastroenterol. 2003;98:1516–24.
35. Fernandez-del Castillo C. Mucinous cystic neoplasms. J Gastrointest Surg. 2008;12:411–3.
36. Fasanella KE, McGrath K. Cystic lesions and intraductal neoplasms of the pancreas. Best Pract Res Clin Gastroenterol. 2009;23:35–48.
37. Genevay M, Mino-Kenudson M, Yaeger K, Konstantinidis IT, Ferrone CR, Thayer S, et al. Cytology adds value to imaging studies for risk assessment of malignancy in pancreatic mucinous cysts. Ann Surg. 2011;254:977–83.
38. Recine M, Kaw M, Evans DB. Fine-needle aspiration cytology of mucinous tumors of the pancreas. Cancer. 2004;102:92–9.
39. Alpert LC, Truong LD, Bossart MI, Spjut HJ. Microcystic adenoma (serous cystadenoma) of the pancreas. A study of 14 cases with immunohistochemical and electron-microscopic correlation. Am J Surg Pathol. 1988;12:251–63.
40. Sarr MG, Murr M, Smyrk TC, Yeo CJ, Fernandez-del-Castillo C, Hawes RH, et al. Primary cystic neoplasms of the pancreas: neoplastic disorders of emerging importance-current state of the art and unanswered questions. J Gastrointest Surg. 2003;7:417–28.
41. Ceppa EP, De la Fuente S, Reddy SK, Stinnett SS, Clary BM, Tyler DS, et al. Defining criteria for selective operative management of pancreatic cystic lesions: does size really matter? J Gastrointest Surg. 2010;14:236–44.
42. Pitman MB. Revised international consensus guidelines for the management of patients with mucinous cysts. Cancer Cytopathol. 2012;120:361–5.
43. Brugge WR, Lewandrowski K, Lee-Lewandrowski E, Centeno BA, Szydlo T, Regan S, et al. Diagnosis of pancreatic cystic neoplasms: a report of the cooperative pancreatic cyst study. Gastroenterology. 2004;126:1330–6.
44. van der Waaij LA, van Dullemen HM, Porte RJ. Cyst fluid analysis in the differential diagnosis of pancreatic cystic lesions: a pooled analysis. Gastrointest Endosc. 2005;62:383–9.
45. Ng DZ, Goh BK, Tham EH, Young SM, Ooi LL. Cystic neoplasms of the pancreas: current diagnostic modalities and management. Ann Acad Med Singapore. 2009;38:251–9.
46. Pais SA, Attasaranya S, Leblanc JK, Sherman S, Schmidt CM, DeWitt J. Role of endoscopic ultrasound in the diagnosis of IPMN: correlation with surgical histopathology. Clin Gastroenterol Hepatol. 2007;5:489–95.
47. Sherman S, et al. Fluid analysis prior to surgical resection of suspected mucinous pancreatic cysts. A single centre experience. J Gastrointest Oncol. 2011;2:208–14.
48. Sakorafas GH, Smyrniotis V, Reid-Lombardo KM, Sarr MG. Primary pancreatic cystic neoplasms revisited: part I: serous cystic neoplasms. Surg Oncol. 2011;20:84–92.
49. Khalid A, McGrath KM, Zahid M, Wilson M, Brody D, Swalsky P, et al. The role of pancreatic cyst fluid molecular analysis in predicting cyst pathology. Clin Gastroenterol Hepatol. 2005;3:967–73.
50. Lee LS, Clancy T, Kadiyala V, Suleiman S, Conwell DL. Interdisciplinary management of cystic neoplasms of the pancreas. Gastroenterol Res Pract. 2012;2:1–7.
51. Khalid A, Zahid M, Finkelstein SD, LeBlanc JK, Kaushik N, Ahmad N, et al. Pancreatic cyst fluid DNA analysis in evaluating pancreatic cysts: a report of the PANDA study. Gastrointest Endosc. 2009;69:1095–102.
52. Chai SM, Herba K, Kumarasinghe MP, de Boer WB, Amanuel B, Grieu-Iacopetta F, et al. Optimizing the multimodal approach to pancreatic cyst fluid diagnosis: developing a volume-based triage protocol. Cancer Cytopathol. 2013;121:86–100.

53. Pitman MB. Pancreatic cyst fluid triage: a critical component of the preoperative evaluation of pancreatic cysts. Cancer Cytopathol. 2013;121:57–60.
54. Schoedel KE, Finkelstein SD, Ohori NP. K-ras and microsatellite marker analysis of fine-needle aspirates from intraductal papillary mucinous neoplasms of the pancreas. Diagn Cytopathol. 2006;34:605–8.
55. O'Toole D, Palazzo L, Arotcarena R, et al. Assessment of complications of EUS-guided fine-needle aspiration. Gastrointest Endosc. 2001;53:470–4.
56. Varadarajulu S, Eloubeidi MA. Frequency and significance of acute intracystic hemorrhage during EUS-FNA of cystic lesions of the pancreas. Gastrointest Endosc. 2004;60:631–5.
57. Hutchins GF, Draganov PV. Cystic neoplasms of the pancreas: a diagnostic challenge. World J Gastroenterol. 2009;15:48–54.
58. Morris-Stiff G, Falk GA, Chalikonda S, Walsh RM. Natural history of asymptomatic pancreatic cystic neoplasms. HPB. 2013;15:175–81.
59. Walsh RM, Zuccaro G, Dumot JA, Vargo J, Biscotti CV, Hammel J, et al. Predicting success of endoscopic aspiration for suspected pancreatic cystic neoplasms. JOP. 2008;9:612–7.
60. Gajoux S, Brennan MF, Gonen M, et al. Cystic lesions of the pancreas: changes in the presentation and management of 1,424 patients at a single institution over a 15-year time period. J Am Coll Surg. 2011;212:590–600.
61. Correa-Gallego C, Ferrone CR, Thayer SP, et al. Incidental pancreatic cysts: do we really know what we are watching? Pancreatology. 2010;10:144–50.
62. Sachs T, Pratt WB, Callery MP, Vollmer Jr CM. The incidental asymptomatic pancreatic lesion: nuisance or threat? J Gastrointest Surg. 2009;13:405–15.
63. Bose D, Tamm E, Liu J, Marcal L, Balachandran A, Bhosale P, et al. Multidisciplinary management strategy for incidental cystic lesions of the pancreas. J Am Coll Surg. 2010;211:205–15.
64. Grobmeyer SR, Cance WG, Copeland EM, Vogel SB, Hochwald SN. Is there an indication for initial conservative management of pancreatic cystic lesions? J Surg Oncol. 2009;100:372–4.
65. Pausawasdi N, Heidt D, Kwon R, Simeone D, Scheiman J. Long-term follow-up of patients with incidentally discovered pancreatic cystic neoplasms evaluated by endoscopic ultrasound. Surgery. 2010;147:13–20.
66. LeBorgne J, de Calan L, Partensky C. Cystadenoma and cystadenocarcinomas of the pancreas: a multiinstitutional retrospective study of 398 cases. French Surgical Association. Ann Surg. 1999;230:152–61.
67. Stelow EB, Bardales RH, Stanley MW. Pitfalls in endoscopic ultrasound-guided fine-needle aspiration and how to avoid them. Adv Anat Pathol. 2005;12:62–73.
68. Al-Haddad M, Gill KR, Raimondo M, Woodward TA, Krishna M, Crook JE, et al. Safety and efficacy of cytology brushings versus standard fine-needle aspiration in evaluating cystic pancreatic lesions: a controlled study. Endoscopy. 2010;42:127–32.
69. Guidelines ASGE. The role of endoscopy in the diagnosis and management of cystic lesions and inflammatory fluid collection of the pancreas. Gastrointest Endosc. 2005;61:363–70.
70. Hong SK, Loren DE, Rogart JN, Siddiqui AA, Sendecki JA, Bibbo M, et al. Targeted cyst wall puncture and aspiration during EUS-FNA increases the diagnostic yield of premalignant and malignant pancreatic cysts. Gastrointest Endosc. 2012;75:775–82.
71. Levy MJ, Smyrk TC, Reddy RP, et al. Endoscopic ultrasound-guided trucut biopsy of the cyst wall for diagnosing cystic pancreatic tumors. Clin Gastroenterol Hepatol. 2005;3:974–9.
72. Sakorafas GH, Mahairas A, Smyrniotis V. Potential pitfalls in the management of primary pancreatic cystic neoplasms. Onkologie. 2011;34:332–6.
73. Salvia R, Malleo G, Marchegiani G, Pennacchio S, Paiella S, Maini M, et al. Pancreatic resections for cystic neoplasms: from the surgeon's presumption to the pathologist's reality. Surgery. 2012;152:S135–42.

Dimitrios Kechagias and Fotios Laspas

5.1 Introduction

The incidental detection of cystic pancreatic lesions has increased with the widespread and frequent use of cross-sectional imaging. Indeed, one or more "cystic lesions" may be noted in up to 27 % of all patients/subjects undergoing modern, state-of-the-art cross-sectional imaging for whatever reason, thereby complicating the job of the radiologist in suggesting who does and who does not need further investigation. Although cystic pancreatic neoplasms are relatively rare medical entity and the vast majority of these cystic "lesions" are benign [1], accurate characterization of a cystic lesion of the pancreas is crucial in determining the appropriate management (imaging follow-up or operative excision). With recent advances in imaging technology, the accuracy of preoperative diagnosis of cystic pancreatic tumors has increased. In many cases, cystic pancreatic neoplasms have characteristic, morphologic imaging features which can suggest or confirm a diagnosis; however, the proper evaluation of these lesions can often be difficult due to morphologic overlap at imaging between benign and malignant tumors.

5.2 Cross-Sectional Imaging (US, CT, MRI)

Cross-sectional imaging modalities remain the mainstay in the detection and assessment of cystic pancreatic tumors. Transabdominal ultrasonography (US) can detect pancreatic cystic lesions; however, given its limited spatial resolution and soft-tissue contrast [2], US is often not very helpful in the evaluation of cystic neoplasms of the pancreas. Multidetector computed tomography (CT) and magnetic resonance imaging (MRI) are the most common radiologic methods used for characterization of

D. Kechagias (✉) • F. Laspas (✉)
CT and MRI Department, Hygeia Hospital, Athens, Greece
e-mail: dikechagias@hotmail.com; fotisdimi@yahoo.gr

© Springer-Verlag Italia 2015   37
G.H. Sakorafas et al. (eds.), *Pancreatic Cystic Neoplasms:*
From Imaging to Differential Diagnosis and Management,
DOI 10.1007/978-88-470-5708-1_5

these lesions. Many authors argue that MRI due to its greater contrast between fluid and soft tissue allows optical depiction of the morphologic features of cystic pancreatic lesions [2, 3]; however, recent studies suggest that both multidetector CT and MRI provide high-quality images of cystic pancreatic lesions with comparable diagnostic accuracy [4, 5]. Although the accuracy of these methods ranges from 40 to 60 % in providing the correct histologic diagnosis of cystic lesions of the pancreas [6], Visser et al. [5] found that multidetector CT and MRI had an accuracy of 76–82 % and 85–91 % respectively in establishing the diagnosis of malignancy in cystic pancreatic masses. The use of advanced MRI techniques, such as diffusion-weighted imaging and ADC measurements, are less helpful currently in distinguishing neoplasmatic from non-neoplasmatic pancreatic cysts than originally hoped [3].

Several important morphologic features of cross-sectional imaging have been shown to be useful in the diagnostic approach to cystic lesions of the pancreas, including the presence of septa (unilocular, oligolocular <6 internal cysts, multilocular ≥6 internal cysts), the size of internal cysts (microcystic <2 cm, macrocystic ≥2 cm), the presence of calcification or mural nodules, and communication of the cystic lesion with the main pancreatic duct [7–9].

Serous cystic neoplasm (SCN) is a benign cystic neoplasm of the pancreas that is more frequently found in older women [2]. The most common pattern (70 % of the cases) of SCN is a lobulated lesion consisting of numerous cysts (more than 6) varying from a few millimeters to 2 cm in diameter (but typically less than 1 cm) [2, 10, 11] (Figs. 5.1 and 5.2). A central fibrous scar that may be calcified is seen up to 30 % of cases and is considered to be characteristic and virtually pathognomonic [9, 10]. Calcification is better depicted on CT (Figs. 5.1 and 5.2). The presence of a large number of very small cysts with innumerable enhancing septa may actually produce what may look like a solid appearance on CT [10–12]. In these cases, clear depiction of numerous discrete small fluid-filled cysts at MRI (due to the high sensitivity of the method in detecting fluid) will usually be diagnostic [10, 12]. Uncommonly, an SCN may have an oligolocular or macrocystic appearance that is difficult to differentiate from other mucinous forms of cystic neoplasms.

Primary mucinous cystic neoplasm (MCN) is found almost exclusively (>90 %) in women (mean age 40–50 years), located typically in the body and tail of the pancreas [1, 13]. Unlike the SCN, the MCN has potential malignancy [13]. A MCN predominantly manifests as a unilocular or mildly septated cystic lesion [2, 14] (Figs. 5.3, 5.4, 5.5, and 5.6). Although the cyst is typically mucin filled, the cystic contents have fluid density on CT, high signal intensity on T2W images, and low signal intensity on T1W images [12]. The internal architecture of the cyst may include papillary projections into the cyst on usually one or more septae [13]. The cyst wall, the septations, and the mural nodules enhance after contrast administration and become more clearly visible [12]. Peripheral calcifications of the cyst are uncommon (<20 %) [13]. In general, mural nodules and septa are better depicted with MRI, whereas calcification is better depicted with CT. Contrary to intraductal papillary mucinous neoplasms (see below), MCNs do not communicate with the pancreatic ductal system. Occasionally, concomitant obstructive pancreatitis may be seen in the distal gland [12, 13]. Peripheral "eggshell" calcification, an irregular

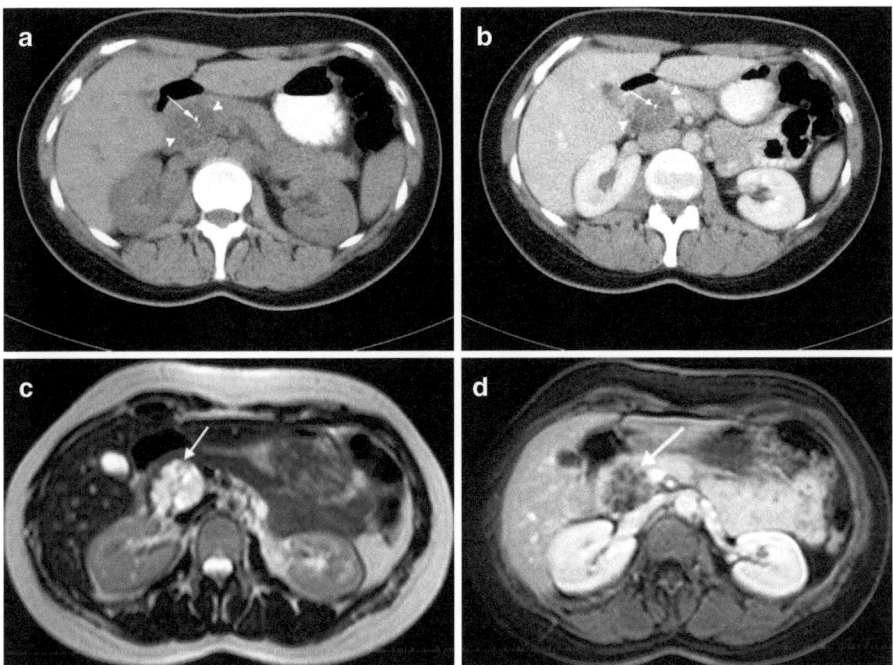

Fig. 5.1 Serous cystic neoplasm. Axial unenhanced (**a**) and contrast-enhanced (**b**) CT images show a lobulated cystic lesion (*arrowheads*) in the pancreatic head with multiple thin internal septation and central calcification (*arrow*). Axial T2-weighted (**c**) and contrast-enhanced T1-weighted (**d**) images of the same patient confirmed the cystic nature of the lesion (*arrow*) consisting of numerous small cysts

wall, thickened septa, papillary projections, an eccentric solid mass, and local invasion of adjacent structures suggest strongly a malignant lesion [13, 14].

Intraductal papillary mucinous neoplasm (IPMN) is a spectrum of related neoplasms characterized by mucinous transformation of the pancreatic ductal epithelium producing an excessive amount of mucin and resulting in dilation of the pancreatic ductal system. IPMN may involve the main pancreatic duct (main-duct type), a side branch off the main duct (branchduct type), or a combination of both (mixed-duct type) (Figs. 5.7, 5.8, and 5.9). The imaging features of IPMN depend on the location of the tumor(s). The main-duct type appears as diffuse or segmental duct dilation [12, 15, 16]. Internal nodular components are best depicted on contrast-enhanced images, but they are usually not seen, because the tumor is small and flat [12, 15]. The branch-duct type appears as a unilocular cystic lesion or as clustered pleomorphic cysts and often involves the uncinate process [15, 16] (Figs. 5.7 and 5.8). The communication between the cystic lesion and the main pancreatic duct is a key feature in the diagnosis [2, 7] (Fig. 5.7c). IPMN may be multifocal and has malignant potential (more likely the main-duct type) [16]. Involvement of the main duct (especially when it is markedly dilated), presence of solid components, diffuse

Fig. 5.2 (**a**) CTs of thick SCNs showing the characteristic microcystic appearance with central calcification (*thick white arrow*) or starburst pattern (*thin white arrow*). (**b**) EUS image demonstrating the classic "honeycombed" microcystic appearance of an SCN (With permission from Fasanella et al. [33])

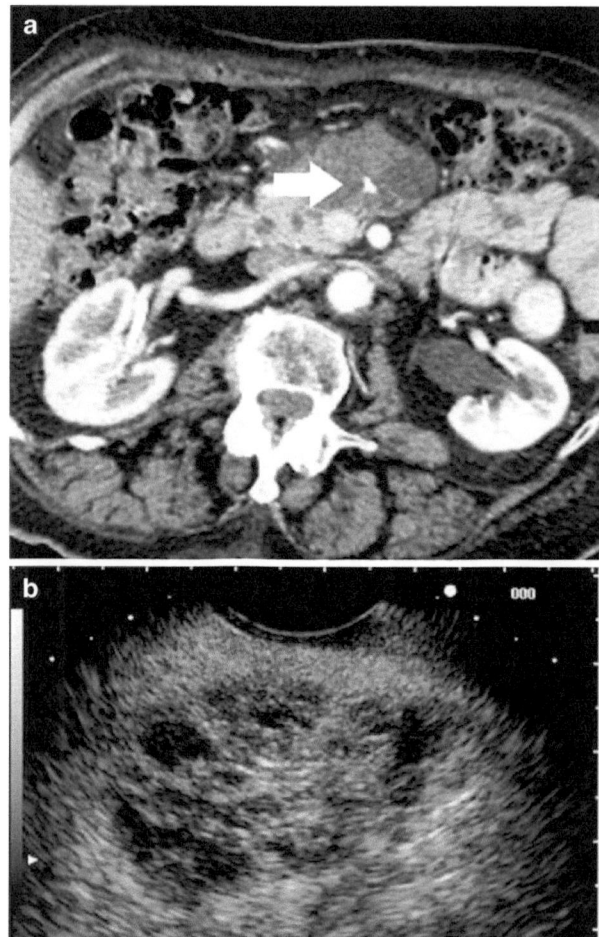

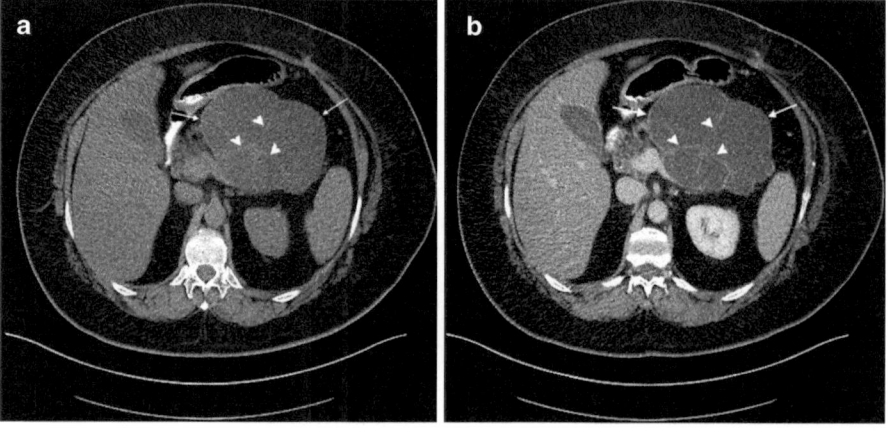

Fig. 5.4 (**a**) CT of a unilocular MCN (*black arrow*) in the pancreatic tail. (**b**) Corresponding EUS image of the mucinous cystic neoplasm, revealing a small septation (*white arrow*) and posterior cyst enhancement (*black arrow*) (Reprinted with permission from Fasanella et al. [33])

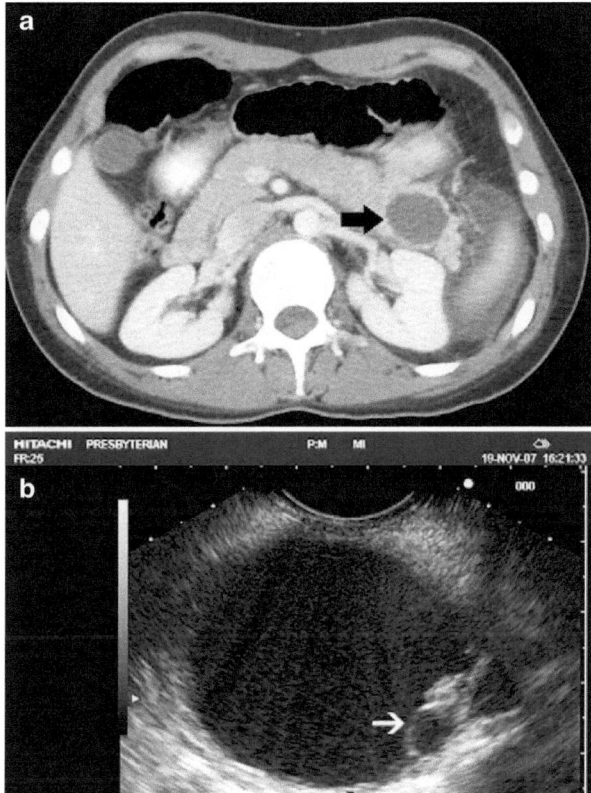

Fig. 5.3 Mucinous cystic neoplasm. Axial unenhanced (**a**) and contrast-enhanced (**b**) CT images show a well-circumscribed cystic lesion (*arrows*) in distal body–tail of pancreas with fine internal septa (*arrowheads*) and multiple cystic foci larger than 1 cm in diameter

Fig. 5.5 Malignant MCNs. (a) Contrast-enhanced CT demonstrating typical cyst wall calcification (*arrowhead*) and enhancing papillary projection (*arrow*). (b) Unenhanced CT shows amorphous calcification of the cyst contents (*arrows*) and incidental large calculus of the collecting system of the left kidney (*arrowhead*) and (c) slightly more caudal image in the same patient as (b) after intravenous contrast medium. Enhancement of the cyst wall demonstrates focal thickening and papillary projection (*arrowhead*) (Reprinted with permission from Scott et al. [34])

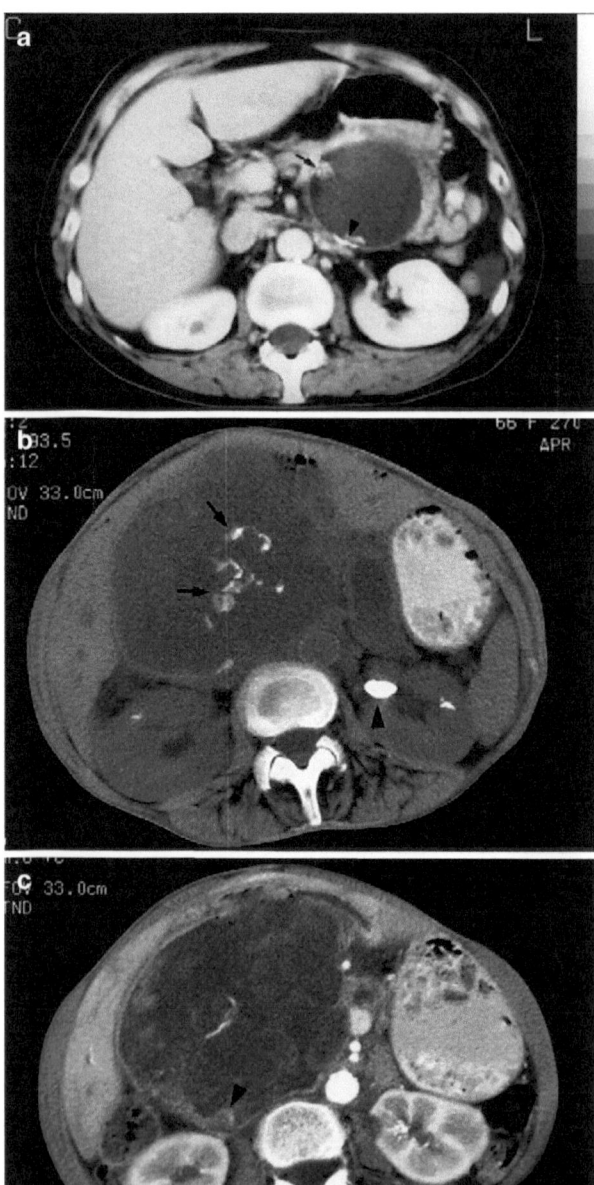

Fig. 5.7 Intraductal papillary mucinous neoplasm, branch duct type. Axial T2-weighted with fat saturation (**a**) and contrast-enhanced T1-weighted (**b**) images depict a pleomorphic cyst (*arrow*) in the uncinate process of the pancreas. Coronal T2-weighted image (**c**) shows communication (*arrow*) between the cyst and the normal caliber main pancreatic duct

Fig. 5.6 CTs of malignant MCN. (**a**) A 69-year-old woman with a large solid/cystic mass encasing the superior mesenteric artery (*arrow*). Multiple cystic liver metastases are seen. (**b**) A 30-year-old woman with a large malignant MCN of the pancreatic tail (*arrowhead*) which has occluded the splenic vein. There are a large wedge-shaped splenic infarct (*thick arrow*) and varices anterior to the spleen (*thin arrow*) (Reprinted with permission from Scott et al. [34])

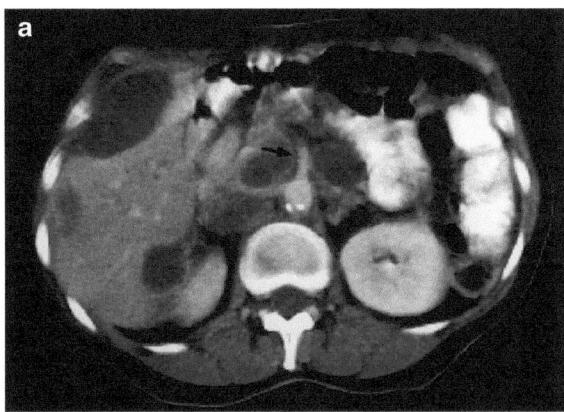

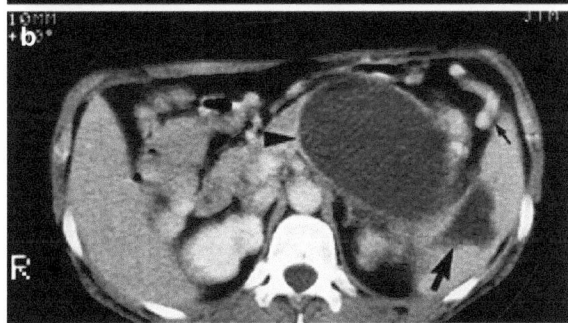

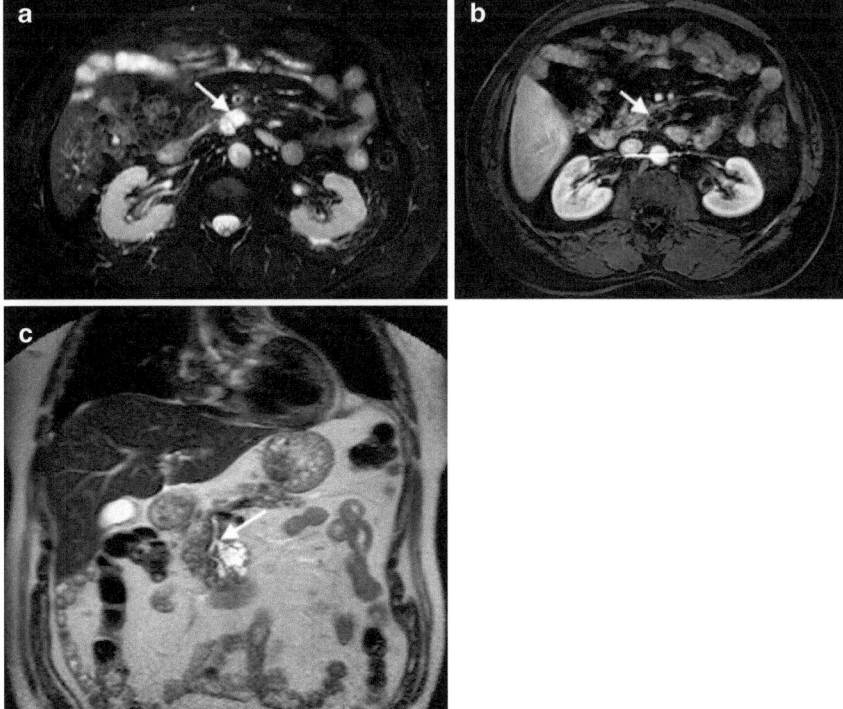

Fig. 5.8 Branch-duct
IPMN. CT shows a 2.5 cm
cystic mass in the uncinate
process (From Katz et al.
[35])

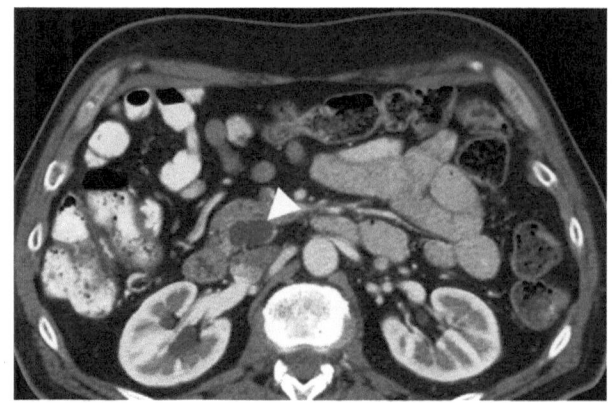

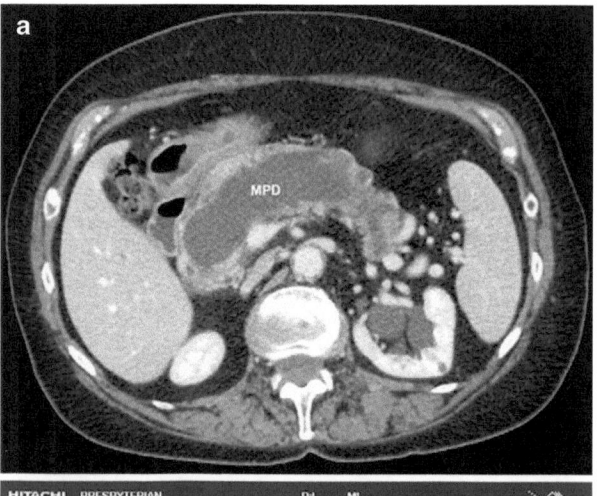

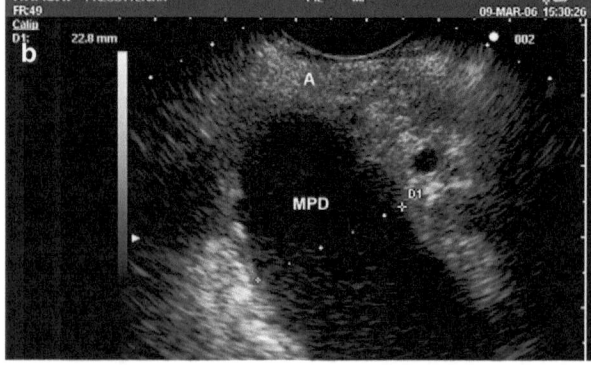

Fig. 5.9 Main-duct IPMN.
(**a**) CT showing marked
dilation of pancreatic duct
and (**b**) EUS of the main
pancreatic duct (*MPD*) of the
patient in Fig. 5.2a (From
Refs. [5, 33])

or multifocal involvement, large size of the lesion, associated biliary obstruction, and extension beyond the gland are signs of malignancy [12, 17].

Solid pseudopapillary tumors, cystic neuroendocrine neoplasms of the pancreas, acinar cell neoplasms, and primary pancreatic adenocarcinomas may on occasion appear as cystic masses. Solid pseudopapillary neoplasm is a rare pancreatic neoplasm that occurs predominantly in young women (<40 years old) and has low malignant potential [2, 18]. CT usually depicts a well-circumscribed lesion with a heterogeneous appearance (mixed solid and cystic components) owing to hemorrhagic degeneration [18, 19]. Calcifications may be present [18]. On MRI images, solid pseudopapillary neoplasms have heterogeneous signal intensity reflecting the complex nature of the mass (Fig. 5.10); moreover, areas of increased signal intensity on T1-weighted images can help identify blood products [18, 19] (Fig. 5.10b). Although pancreatic neuroendocrine neoplasms are typically solid and hypervascular masses, marked cystic changes may be seen [2, 20]. Imaging reveals typically a thick-walled cystic lesion, and the presence of hypervascular tissue that enhances avidly in the arterial phase suggests the diagnosis [2, 12]. Primary pancreatic adenocarcinomas and acinar cell neoplasms may rarely develop areas of cystic degeneration and necrosis (usually when they are large in size) and resemble other cystic pancreatic neoplasms [1, 6].

5.3   Endoscopic Ultrasonography (EUS)

EUS has emerged as a very valuable tool for characterizing cystic pancreatic lesions. Internal positioning of the probe allows close proximity between the transducer and the cystic pancreatic lesion providing greater resolution images for a very precise definition of the cyst morphology [6, 21]. As with CT and MRI, EUS is capable of defining cystic localization, size, locularity, mural nodules, cystic wall, calcifications, and communication between the pancreatic duct and cyst. The typical

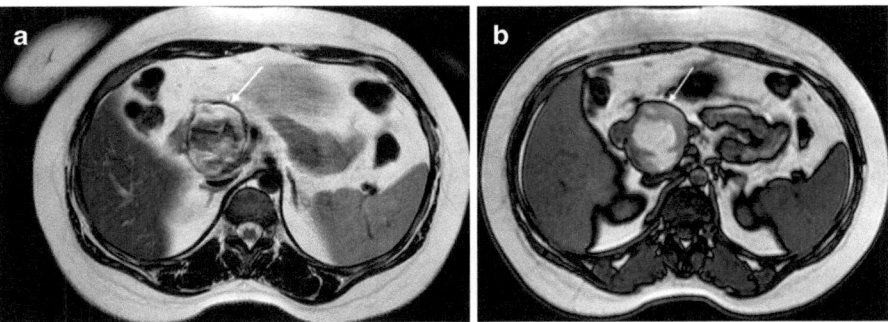

Fig. 5.10 Solid pseudopapillary tumor. (**a**) Axial T2-weighted image demonstrates a well-circumscribed mass (*arrow*) in the head of the pancreas with complex internal signal intensity. (**b**) Axial unenhanced T1-weighted image depicts regions of high signal intensity within the mass (*arrow*), which represent blood products from hemorrhagic degeneration

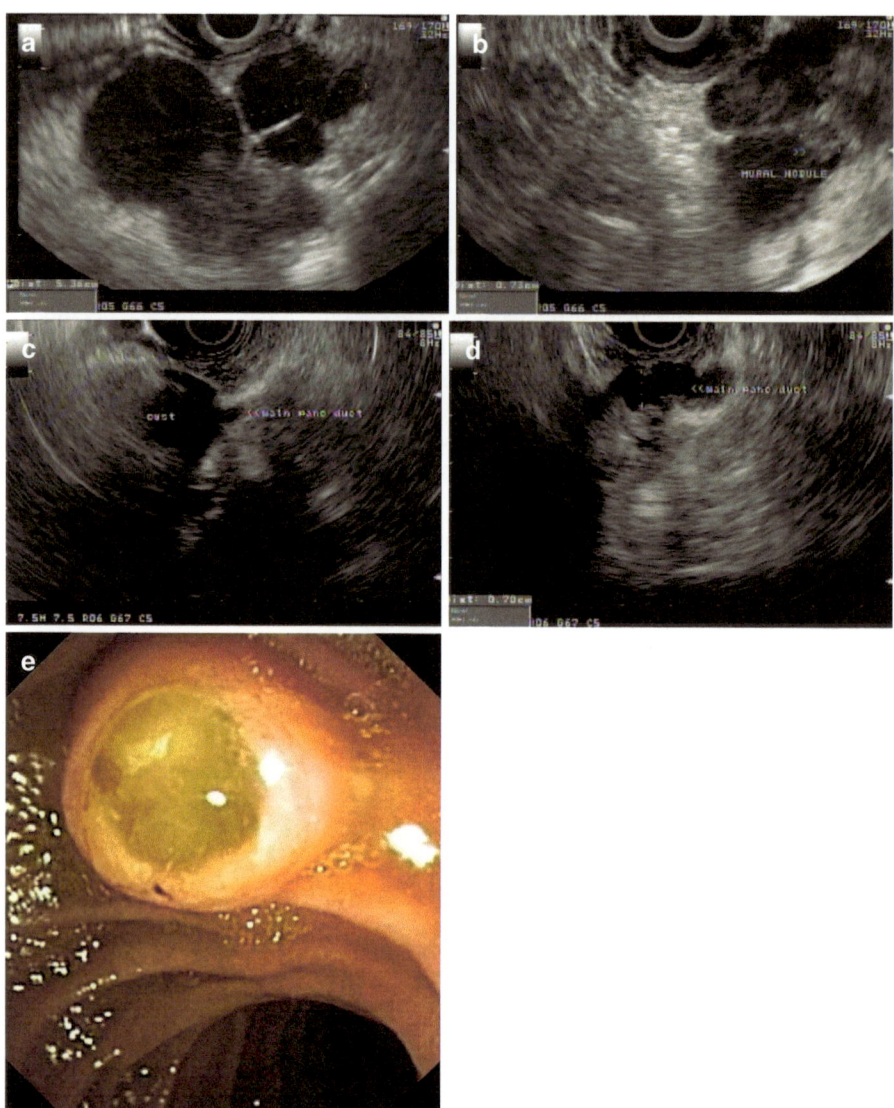

Fig. 5.11 Intraductal papillary mucinous neoplasm, mixed-duct type. Endoscopic ultrasonography reveals a complex pancreatic cystic mass (**a**) with hyperechoic mural nodule (**b**), communication between the lesion and the main pancreatic duct (**c**), and dilation of the pancreatic duct (**d**). Endoscopic view (**e**) of the same patient shows an expanded papilla of Vater with egress of mucous, a finding that supports strongly the diagnosis of an IPMN

microcystic SCN with possible calcification of the central fibrous scar is well seen on EUS [6, 10]. On EUS, MCNs are typically a unilocular anechoic or macrocystic lesion in the body or the tail of the pancreas, and criteria for malignancy (peripheral calcification, an irregular wall, thickened septa, eccentric mass, and papillary projections) can be detected [6, 13]. Findings of IPMN on EUS include diffuse or segmental dilation of the pancreatic duct (main-duct type), a unilocular or a clustered cystic lesion (branch-duct type), communication between pancreatic cystic lesions and the pancreatic duct, and mural nodules as isoechoic or hyperechoic papillary projection of the duct wall [6, 16] (Fig. 5.11).

A wide range of diagnostic accuracy of EUS morphology in differentiating cystic lesions of the pancreas has been reported (results of between 51 and 90 %) [21]. There are few studies comparing the accuracy of radiologic techniques (CT and MRI) and EUS in pancreatic cystic lesions. Gerke et al. [22] found that EUS and CT are similarly accurate in the characterization of cystic pancreatic lesions as benign or malignant (66 % for EUS and 71 % for CT with very poor agreement between them). More recent studies [23, 24] reported equivalent diagnostic performance between EUS and MRI to differentiate malignant from benign cystic pancreatic lesions. However, Kim et al. [24] found that interobserver agreement was better on MRI than EUS, because EUS is a highly operator-dependent technique.

5.4 Magnetic Resonance Cholangiopancreatography (MRCP)

MRCP is a noninvasive diagnostic method which utilizes the inherent contrast of the fluid-filled ducts to generate images of the biliary system and pancreatic duct. It is based on a heavily T2-weighted pulse sequence which shows static or slow-moving fluid-filled structures, such as the bile and pancreatic ducts, appearing at greatly high signal intensity, whereas the surrounding structures generate little signal resulting in increased duct-to-background contrast. MRCP provides excellent depiction of the pancreatic duct (Fig. 5.12) allowing the identification of even a small communication between a pancreatic cystic lesion and the pancreatic ductal system [2]; this finding on MRCP can on occasion be more specific than ERCP, because filling of side branch ducts at the time of ERCP may be obscured by intraductal plugs of mucus [16]. Thereby, MRCP may be helpful in differentiating a primary MCN of the pancreas from a branch-duct-type IPMN by showing the absence or presence, respectively, of a ductal communication [13]. Moreover, internal nodular components in a main-duct-type IPMN as well as concomitant side branch lesions of IPMN may be detected on MRCP [16].

5.5 Other Imaging Modalities

Endoscopic retrograde cholangiopancreatography (ERCP) is a very sensitive method to reveal the communication between a pancreatic cystic lesion and the pancreatic ductal system, a finding which is indicative of a pseudocyst or an IPMN [13, 25], but ERCP is invasive. In IPMN, ERCP can demonstrate clearly segmental or diffuse dilation of the main pancreatic duct that may contain filling defects caused by mucus or related to mural nodular lesions [16, 25] (Figs. 5.13 and 5.14). Filling defects caused

Fig. 5.12 Intraductal
papillary mucinous neoplasm,
mixed-duct type. Single-slice
MRCP image shows a
multilocular cystic lesion
(*arrows*) in the pancreatic
body and dilation of the main
pancreatic duct (*arrowheads*)

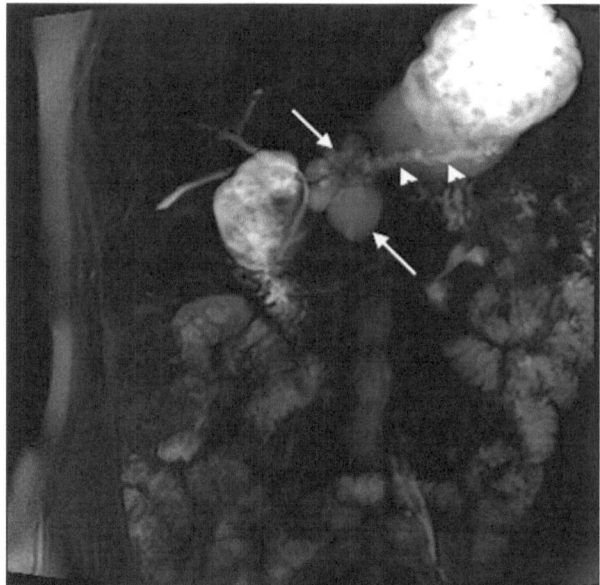

Fig. 5.13 Imaging of
intraductal "masses." ERCP
of main-duct IPMN with
multiple filling defects
secondary to mucinous
globules (From Sarr et al.
[36])

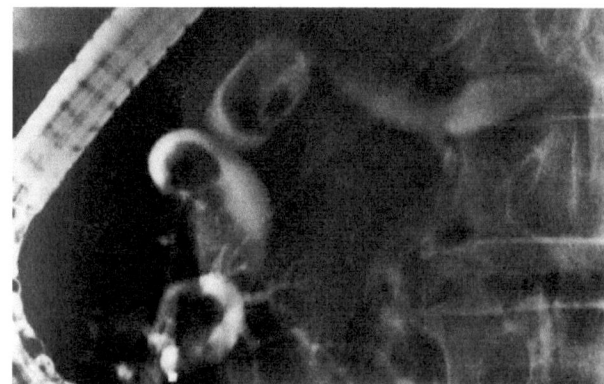

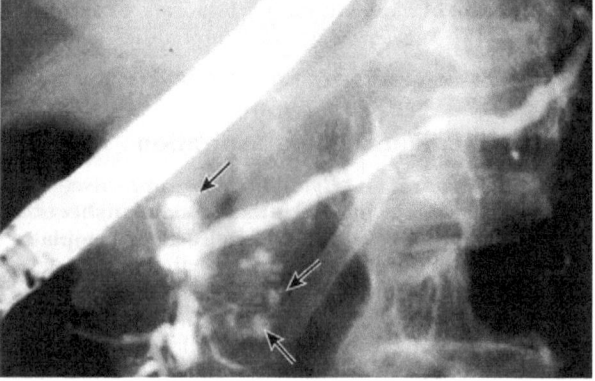

Fig. 5.14 ERCPs showing
communication with cystic
areas in branch-duct
IPMN (uncinate and head of
pancreas) (From Sarr et al.
[36])

by mucus may be moved when passed with a catheter or a guidewire, while persistent filling defects probably represent papillary neoplasms [25]. A finding on ERCP that supports strongly the diagnosis of an IPMN is the recognition of a bulging ampulla of Vater with extrusion of mucus; this pathognomonic finding is seen in 30 % of patients with main-duct- or mixed-duct-type IPMN (Fig. 5.15) [16, 25]. Pancreatic ductal brushings can be also retrieved during ERCP for analysis and cytology. However, due to the considerable advances of noninvasive imaging modalities, the cost, and because ERCP is invasive, the use of ERCP for solely diagnostic purposes is declining.

Positron emission tomography (PET) has a potential advantage in the detection of malignant lesions, because PET provides "functional" information. Hybrid PET/CT combines the functional data of PET with the anatomic details of CT. Although the role of PET in the evaluation of various other solid pancreatic tumors is established, its role in cystic pancreatic neoplasms is still evolving. False-negative results for borderline and noninvasive malignant neoplasms remain a major limitation of PET in the evaluation of pancreatic cystic lesions [13]. A prospective study [26] showed that PET was highly accurate in distinguishing benign and malignant IPMNs with a specificity and sensitivity of 92 % and 97 %, respectively. Hong et al. [27] found that PET/CT outperformed multidetector CT alone in the characterization of malignant IPMNs. Despite the potential added benefits of PET, the published studies have shown that the limitations of conventional images in discriminating borderline and noninvasive neoplasms cannot be overcome by PET [28]. Moreover, PET is much more expensive and may not provide further information worth the considerably added cost of PET. More studies are needed in order to determine the role of PET in the management of pancreatic cystic lesions.

Intraductal pancreatoscopy can be performed in selected centers. The introduction of a small-diameter endoscope (under duodenoscopic assistance) into the pancreatic duct can provide direct visualization of the ductal epithelium (Fig. 5.16). Recently, the method has been combined with narrowband imaging emphasizing certain image features, such as mucosal structures and capillary vessels [29]. Intraductal ultrasonography using high-frequency ultrasound probes during ERCP

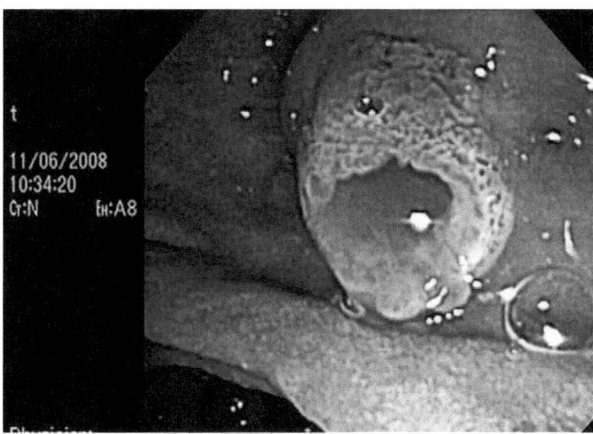

Fig 5.15 Endoscopic view of bulging papilla of Vater with egress of copious mucous (From Refs. [37])

Fig. 5.16 Peroral
pancreatoscopic photograph
showing a fish egg-like
mucosal lesion in the main
pancreatic duct in a patient
with IPMN (From Tanaka
et al. [38])

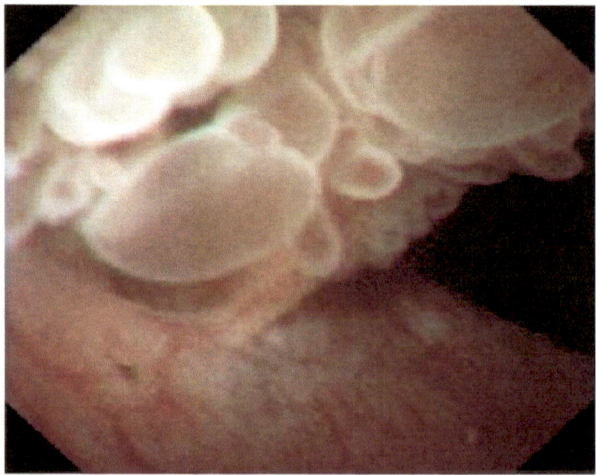

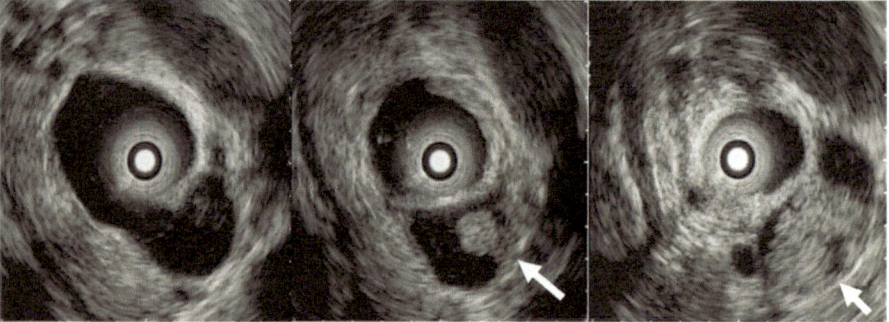

Fig. 5.17 Intraductal ultrasonogram visualizing a mural nodule in a branch-duct IPMN in the head of the pancreas (*arrows*) (From Tanaka et al. [38])

enables the examination of the main pancreatic duct and surrounding structures (Fig. 5.17). Currently, IPMN is considered the most suitable indication of these newer diagnostic techniques, because they may be useful for diagnosing and distinguishing benign from malignant IPMN [29–32]. Although the results are very promising, the lack of availability and the use of these modalities to only a few selected centers remains a noteworthy limitation.

References

1. Acar M, Tatli S. Cystic tumors of the pancreas: a radiological perspective. Diagn Interv Radiol. 2011;17:143–9.
2. Kalb B, Sarmiento JM, Kooby DA, Adsay NV, Martin DR. MR imaging of cystic lesions of the pancreas. Radiographics. 2009;29:1749–65.

3. Wang Y, Miller FH, Chen ZE, Merrick L, Mortele KJ, Hoff FL, Hammond NA, Yaghmai V, Nikolaidis P. Diffusion-weighted MR imaging of solid and cystic lesions of the pancreas. Radiographics. 2011;31:47–64.
4. Sahani DV, Kambadakone A, Macari M, Takahashi N, Chari S, Fernandez-del Castillo C. Diagnosis and management of cystic pancreatic lesions. AJR Am J Roentgenol. 2013;200:343–54.
5. Visser BC, Yeh BM, Qayyum A, Way LW, Mc-Culloch CE, Coakley FV. Characterization of cystic pancreatic masses: relative accuracy of CT and MRI. AJR Am J Roentgenol. 2007; 189:648–56.
6. Kucera JN, Kucera S, Perrin SD, Caracciolo JT, Schmulewitz N, Kedar RP. Cystic lesions of the pancreas: radiologic-endosonographic correlation. Radiographics. 2012;32:283–301.
7. Ng DZ, Goh BK, Tham EH, Young SM, Ooi LL. Cystic neoplasms of the pancreas: current diagnostic modalities and management. Ann Acad Med Singapore. 2009;38:251–9.
8. Sahani DV, Kadavigere R, Saokar A, Fernandez-del Castillo C, Brugge WR, Hahn PF. Cystic pancreatic lesions: a simple imaging-based classification system for guiding management. Radiographics. 2005;25:1471–84.
9. Macari M, Megibow AJ. Focal cystic pancreatic lesions: variability in radiologists' recommendations for follow-up imaging. Radiology. 2011;259:20–3.
10. Sakorafas GH, Smyrniotis V, Reid-Lombardo KM, Sarr MG. Primary pancreatic cystic neoplasms revisited. Part I: serous cystic neoplasms. Surg Oncol. 2011;20:84–92.
11. Kim YH, Saini S, Sahani D, Hahn PF, Mueller PR, Auh YH. Imaging diagnosis of cystic pancreatic lesions: pseudocyst versus nonpseudocyst. Radiographics. 2005;25:671–85.
12. Khan A, Khosa F, Eisenberg RL. Cystic lesions of the pancreas. AJR. 2011;196:668–77.
13. Sakorafas GH, Smyrniotis V, Reid-Lombardo KM, Sarr MG. Primary pancreatic cystic neoplasms revisited: part II. Mucinous cystic neoplasms. Surg Oncol. 2011;20:93–101.
14. Testini M, Gurrado A, Lissidini G, Venezia P, Greco L, Piccinni G. Management of mucinous cystic neoplasms of the pancreas. World J Gastroenterol. 2010;16:5682–92.
15. Lim JH, Lee G, Oh YL. Radiologic spectrum of intraductal papillary mucinous tumor of the pancreas. Radiographics. 2001;21:323–37.
16. Sakorafas GH, Smyrniotis V, Reid-Lombardo KM, Sarr MG. Primary pancreatic cystic neoplasms revisited. Part III. Intraductal papillary mucinous neoplasms. Surg Oncol. 2011;20:109–18.
17. Kawamoto S, Horton KM, Lawler LP, Hruban RH, Fishman EK. Intraductal papillary mucinous neoplasm of the pancreas: can benign lesions be differentiated from malignant lesions with multidetector CT? Radiographics. 2005;25:1451–68.
18. Choi JY, Kim MJ, Kim JH, Kim SH, Lim JS, Oh YT, Chung JJ, Yoo HS, Lee JT, Kim KW. Solid pseudopapillary tumor of the pancreas: typical and atypical manifestations. AJR. 2006;187:178–86.
19. Coleman KM, Doherty MC, Bigler SA. Solid-pseudopapillary tumor of the pancreas. Radiographics. 2003;23:1644–8.
20. Sakorafas GH, Smyrniotis V, Reid-Lombardo KM, Sarr MG. Primary pancreatic cystic neoplasms of the pancreas revisited. Part IV: rare cystic neoplasms. Surg Oncol. 2012;21:153–63.
21. Barresi L, Tarantino I, Granata A, Curcio G, Traina M. Pancreatic cystic lesions: How endoscopic ultrasound morphology and endoscopic ultrasound fine needle aspiration help unlock the diagnostic puzzle. World J Gastrointest Endosc. 2012;4:247–59.
22. Gerke H, Jaffe TA, Mitchell RM, Byrne MF, Stiffler HL, Branch MS, Baillie J, Jowell PS. Endoscopic ultrasound and computer tomography are inaccurate methods of classifying cystic pancreatic lesions. Dig Liver Dis. 2006;38:39–44.
23. Kim YC, Choi JY, Chung YE, Bang S, Kim MJ, Park MS, Kim KW. Comparison of MRI and endoscopic ultrasound in the characterization of pancreatic cystic lesions. AJR. 2010;195:947–52.
24. Kim JH, Eun HW, Park HJ, Hong SS, Kim YJ. Diagnostic performance of MRI and EUS in the differentiation of benign from malignant pancreatic cyst and cyst communication with the main duct. Eur J Radiol. 2012;81:2927–35.

25. Jacobson BC, Baron TH, Adler DG, Davila RE, Egan J, Hirota WK, Leighton JA, Qureshi W, Rajan E, Zuckerman MJ, Fanelli R, Wheeler-Harbaugh J, Faigel DO. ASGE guideline: the role of endoscopy in the diagnosis and the management of cystic lesions and inflammatory fluid collections of the pancreas. Gastrointest Endosc. 2005;61:363–70.
26. Sperti C, Bissoli S, Pasquali C, Frison L, Liessi G, Chierichetti F, Pedrazzoli S. 18-fluorodeoxyglucose positron emission tomography enhances computed tomography diagnosis of malignant intraductal papillary mucinous neoplasms of the pancreas. Ann Surg. 2007;246:932–7.
27. Hong HS, Yun M, Cho A, Choi JY, Kim MJ, Kim KW, Choi YJ, Lee JD. The utility of F-18 FDG PET/CT in the evaluation of pancreatic intraductal papillary mucinous neoplasm. Clin Nucl Med. 2010;35:776–9.
28. Sahani DV, Bonaffini PA, Catalano OA, Guimaraes AR, Blake MA. State-of-the-art PET/CT of the pancreas: current role and emerging indications. Radiographics. 2012;32:1133–58.
29. Itoi T, Sofuni A, Itokawa F, Kurihara T, Tsuchiya T, Ishii K, Tsuji S, Ikeuchi N, Arisaka Y, Moriyasu F. Initial experience of peroral pancreatoscopy combined with narrow-band imaging in the diagnosis of intraductal papillary mucinous neoplasms of the pancreas (with videos). Gastrointest Endosc. 2007;66:793–7.
30. Hara T, Yamaguchi T, Ishihara T, Tsuyuguchi T, Kondo F, Kato K, Asano T, Saisho H. Diagnosis and patient management of intraductal papillary-mucinous tumor of the pancreas by using peroral pancreatoscopy and intraductal ultrasonography. Gastroenterology. 2002;122:34–43.
31. Yasuda K, Sakata M, Ueda M, Uno K, Nakajima M. The use of pancreatoscopy in the diagnosis of intraductal papillary mucinous tumor lesions of the pancreas. Clin Gastroenterol Hepatol. 2005;3:53–7.
32. Turner BG, Brugge WR. Diagnostic and therapeutic endoscopic approaches to intraductal papillary mucinous neoplasm. World J Gastrointest Surg. 2010;2:337–41. 27.
33. Fasanella KE, et al. Cystic lesions and intraductal neoplasms of the pancreas. Best Pract Res Clin Gastroenterol. 2009;23:35–48.
34. Scott J, et al. Mucinous cystic neoplasms of the pancreas: Imaging features and diagnostic difficulties. Clin Radiol. 2000;55:187–92.
35. Katz MH, et al. Diagnosis and management of cystic neoplasms of the pancreas: an evidence-based approach. J Am Coll Surg. 2008;207:106–20.
36. Sarr MG, et al. Primary cystic neoplasms of the pancreas. Neoplastic disorders of emerging importance. J Gastrointest Surg. 2003;7:417–28.
37. Roggin KK, et al. Pancreatic cystic neoplasm. Curr Probl Surg. 2010;47:459–510.
38. Tanaka M, et al. International consensus guidelines for management of intraductal papillary mucinous neoplasms and mucinous cystic neoplasms of the pancreas. Pancreatology. 2006;6(1–2):17–32.

Treatment of Pancreatic Cystic Neoplasms

6

George H. Sakorafas, Vassileios Smyrniotis,
and Michael G. Sarr

Therapeutic decision-making in patients with PCNs depends on multiple factors, including presenting symptoms, the general status of the patient (presence of clinically relevant comorbidities, age, etc.), and in large part the morphologic features on cross-sectional imaging. Currently, preoperative diagnosis and identification of characteristics indicating malignant disease or premalignant potential are possible with an overall accuracy of about 70 %, mainly as a result of the increasing awareness and recent technical progress in imaging modalities [2].

Operative resection is the cornerstone in the management of PCNs. Resection may achieve cure and long-term survival, relief of symptoms, and diagnostic certainty [3]. Pancreatectomy, however (and in particular pancreatic head resection), is associated with a low but still substantial mortality (~2 %) and a high morbidity (~40–50 %), even in high-volume centers. In the process of decision-making concerning therapy, the risk of undertreatment of a premalignant or malignant cystic neoplasm needs to be weighed carefully against the risk (morbidity/mortality) of pancreatic resection. The identification of selected subgroups of patients in whom a more conservative approach might be appropriate has attracted the interest of many investigators around the world.

G.H. Sakorafas, MD (✉)
Department of Surgical Oncology, Saint Savvas Cancer Hospital,
Arkadias 19-21, Athens 11526, Greece
e-mail: georgesakorafas@yahoo.com

V. Smyrniotis, MD
4th Department of Surgery, Attikon University Hospital, Chanioti 22, Athens 15452, Greece
e-mail: vsmyrniotis@hotmail.com

M.G. Sarr, MD
Department of Surgery, Mayo Clinic, 200 First Street SW, Rochester, MN 55905, USA
e-mail: sarr.michael@mayo.edu

© Springer-Verlag Italia 2015
G.H. Sakorafas et al. (eds.), *Pancreatic Cystic Neoplasms:
From Imaging to Differential Diagnosis and Management*,
DOI 10.1007/978-88-470-5708-1_6

6.1   Serous Cystic Neoplasms

6.1.1   Indications for Resection

Given that malignant transformation of SCNs is extremely rare (risk, 0–1.2 %) [4–8], a conservative approach of surveillance imaging has been proposed as a logical therapeutic strategy [8–11]. This strategy remains a bit controversial, however, and has been challenged recently. The decrease in perioperative mortality after major pancreatic resections observed during the last two decades may account in part for the change of treatment policy toward a more aggressive approach with resection recommended for most (or even all) cystic neoplasms involving the body or tail of the pancreas [12, 13]. The rare but recently described "locally aggressive" SCN (which is characterized by local invasion, occurring in 5 % of patients) supports an aggressive approach of treatment; this subtype of unusual SCNs manifests an aggressive behavior, defined as local involvement of surrounding strictures (bile/pancreatic duct, extrahepatic venous system, etc.), and has the potential of distant (hepatic) metastases [7]. A conservative approach, however, can be considered in the vast majority of patients with SCN (e.g., in the presence of a small, asymptomatic lesion in the pancreatic head, especially in a frail or elderly patient), given the slow progression of these lesions over many years [14–16]. Indeed, in the study by Bassi et al. [17], 50 patients with SCN who were managed non-operatively had no evidence of a "significant increase in the diameter of the lesion" after a median follow-up of 69 months. In contrast, Tseng et al. [8], from the Massachusetts General Hospital, reported their experience with 24 of 106 patients with SCNs followed longitudinally over time and found a rate of growth of 0.6 cm/year. Growth rate was correlated with initial tumor size (0.12 cm/year in tumors <4 cm in size [$n=15$ patients] vs. 1.98 cm/year in tumors ≥ 4 cm [$n=9$ patients], $p=0.0002$). This information regarding the natural history of untreated SCNs has relevant clinical importance. Although it remains unclear whether this increased rate of growth in the larger SCNs has any impact on malignant potential [12], an increased growth rate intuitively would increase the risk of the SCNs becoming symptomatic within the lifetime of many patients. Indeed, large (≥ 4 cm) SCNs are associated with a more than threefold increase in the likelihood of developing symptoms [8].

Currently, the accepted indications for operative intervention in patients with SCNs include [8, 14, 18, 19]:

1. Presence of relevant symptomatology, which is usually due to local compression (not invasion) of surrounding structures.
2. Size ≥ 4 cm.
3. Rapid enlargement of a SCN or presence of an eccentric mass or pericystic infiltrative appearance such as biliary or pancreatic ductal obstruction (findings raising concerns about the presence of malignancy).
4. Uncertainty about the type of cystic neoplasm (SCN vs. MCN), despite the use of modern and sophisticated diagnostic tools (see above). Indeed, as sensitivity for the diagnosis of the potentially malignant mucinous neoplasms increases, the specificity decreases. When a preoperative diagnosis cannot be established with

a reasonable level of confidence, resection should be considered strongly. In this case, resection is often performed to avoid potential undertreatment of an otherwise curable overt or premalignant neoplasm.

6.1.2   Type of Resection

Anatomic pancreatic resection depending on the location of the SCN is the procedure of choice. If the SCN is located in the pancreatic head, pancreatoduodenectomy (preferentially with pylorus preservation) is indicated [3]. From a technical point of view, it should be noted that pancreatoduodenectomy in the setting of a SCN, in contrast to pancreatic ductal adenocarcinoma, will often be complicated by the presence of a normal, soft pancreatic parenchyma and non-dilated pancreatic and biliary ducts [20]. For SCNs located in the distal pancreas (body/tail), distal pancreatectomy (typically with or without splenectomy) is usually required [14, 19]. Other tissue-preserving procedures, such as segmental "central" pancreatectomy, duodenum-preserving pancreatic head resection, or even enucleation, have been described [19, 21]; however, when selecting these procedures, caution is required when the preoperative diagnosis is not secure. Specifically regarding enucleation, it should be noted that – in some studies – it is associated with a high morbidity (up to 35 %), mainly due to the occurrence of postoperative pancreatic fistula [13]; moreover, enucleation is often not a realistic option because of the large size and location of the neoplasm. There is no role for total pancreatectomy, lymphadenectomy, or "extended" resection in the management of SCNs.

6.2   Mucinous Cystic Neoplasms

6.2.1   Indications for Resection

As noted above and in contrast to SCNs, MCNs represent a more diverse, heterogeneous spectrum of biologic behavior, compatible with the classic model of carcinogenesis with progression from atypia to dysplasia to *carcinoma* in situ and (potentially) to invasive malignancy as seen in many other cancers. Therefore, MCNs are considered to be potentially premalignant and as such can undergo malignant degeneration at any time [9, 10, 14]; the whole spectrum of neoplasia (multicentric metaplasia, dysplasia, carcinoma in situ, and invasive carcinoma) may coexist within the same neoplasm [9, 10]. Malignant degeneration of a MCN appears to be relatively common and has been described, often presumably taking a long period of time (years) to develop [22]. Risk factors indicating the presence of malignancy include [9, 22, 23, 25, 26]:

1. Large tumor size: Goh et al. reported that none of the 40 malignant MCNs (carcinoma in situ or invasive) were <3 cm, and only one was <4.5 cm (3 cm) [25]. In the study by Crippa et al. of 163 resected MCNs, all neoplasms with cancer

Table 6.1 Sendai recommendations of the International Association of Pancreatology regarding management of IPMNs and MCNs

MD-IPMNs
Ideally, all main-duct and mixed variant IPMNs should be resected (in patients who are good surgical candidates with reasonable life expectancy)
BD-IPMN
Resection is indicated in the presence of symptoms or risk factors for malignancy (presence of mural nodules and cyst size >3 cm)
Patients with small cysts without other risk factors can be treated conservatively. Decision to treat operatively should be individualized
MCNs
Resection is always indicated, unless there are contraindications for operation

Modified from Tanaka et al. [35]

were ≥4 cm, and malignant MCNs (carcinoma in situ and invasive) were larger than benign ones (8 cm vs. 4.5 cm). Moreover, a diameter ≥6 cm was associated with a much greater risk for malignancy [24].

2. Associated eccentric solid mass, mural nodules, mixed solid and cystic components, marked papillary projections, an asymmetrically thickened wall or irregularity of borders, hypervascularity, etc. Malignant MCNs (both in situ and invasive carcinoma) were 16 times more likely to harbor nodules (64 % vs. 4 %). Moreover, all MCNs with cancer were either ≥4 cm in size or had nodules [24].

3. Calcifications (often peripheral, eggshell-like).

4. Age. Patients with invasive carcinoma were older (55 vs. 44 years) than those with noninvasive MCNs.

Because of their malignant potential, resection in the good risk patient is considered as the treatment of choice for most MCNs, provided that the operative risk is acceptable [9, 10, 22, 24, 26]. This aggressive approach is supported by the recent (2012) consensus guidelines of the International Association of Pancreatology (Table 6.1).

A conservative approach of serial surveillance imaging has been proposed recently by some groups in patients with presumably low-risk MCN (i.e., asymptomatic MCNs, size <3 cm, no mural nodules, and no pancreatic or common bile duct dilation) [24, 26–28]. This approach of "watchful waiting" represents a trade-off between the potential of delaying resection with future development of unresectable disease and any unnecessary operative morbidity and mortality with early resection for benign MCNs. A planned watchful surveillance could be considered in high-risk patients with severe comorbidity or in the elderly [23], as suggested by the recent IAP consensus guidelines (Table 6.1). The patient should be well informed about the risks associated with a conservative approach and understand that even today, with the availability of modern, sophisticated diagnostic methods, accurate preoperative detection of malignancy within most MCNs is not possible [23].

6.2.2 Types of Resections

Because of the malignant potential of MCNs and the uncertainty which exists pre-operatively or even intraoperatively about the presence of malignant degeneration, a formal, oncologic, radical anatomic pancreatectomy (depending on the location of the neoplasm) is indicated. Pancreatoduodenectomy (preferentially with pylorus preservation) should be performed for MCNs located in the pancreatic head, while MCNs located in the distal pancreas (which is the most common location of MCNs) are treated by distal pancreatectomy and splenectomy. Given that distal pancreatectomy is easier and safer compared to pancreatoduodenectomy, the decision to proceed to pancreatic resection for MCN in the body/tail of the pancreas is an easier decision for both patient and surgeon compared to lesions of the pancreatic head, which require pancreatoduodenectomy, a procedure associated with much greater morbidity and mortality. A laparoscopic approach is an acceptable alternative for small- or even medium-sized MCNs located in the body or tail of the pancreas [29]. It is important not to rupture the cyst during the procedure, because spillage of its contents could lead potentially to tumor spread. Moreover, the cyst should be removed intact (i.e., not morselized) so the pathologist can do an appropriate (and complete) examination. Spleen preservation may be reasonable in small- or medium-sized lesions without any findings suggestive of malignancy [30].

Less extensive resections, such as segmental "central" pancreatectomy or distal pancreatectomy with spleen preservation, offer the advantage of preserving functional pancreatic parenchyma and thereby potentially avoiding insulin-dependent diabetes. These types of parenchyma-preserving resections could be considered in small MCNs (<4 cm) and when there are no indications that the neoplasm has an invasive component (2012 IAP consensus guidelines) [31]; yet, this decision is taken with a small calculated risk (<10 %) of treating an invasive malignancy without the ideal oncologic extent of resection [22]. Lesser, nonanatomic resections, such as enucleation or duodenum-preserving, subtotal resection of the pancreatic head, although feasible technically, appear to be suboptimal procedures, given the limitations in preoperative and intraoperative diagnosis of invasive carcinoma [1, 32].

Excision of lymph nodes beyond those immediately adjacent to the pancreas is not necessary or beneficial, even when there is a high suspicion of malignancy, because the incidence of lymph node metastases in malignant MCNs is relatively low [24, 30]. Rarely, resection of involved adjacent structures/organs (including portal vein) may be required; however, unlike pancreatic adenocarcinomas, malignant MCNs tend to be "pushers" rather than "invaders" [33].

Frozen-section analysis of operative margins as is done with IPMN is not required during operation for MCNs, because cyst boundaries are easily discernible. Results of frozen-section analysis in an attempt to differentiate MCN from pseudocyst (and thereby determine operative procedure – resection vs. enteric drainage) may be misleading, because MCNs frequently have an incomplete, discontinuous epithelial liming and may be indistinguishable from a pseudocyst on cursory frozen section [9, 14, 26, 34]. Frozen-section analysis may be indicated to exclude invasive malignancy if a dubious firmness is close to the resection margin. If invasive carcinoma is detected at the margin, a more extensive resection designed to obtain negative margins should be undertaken as for any other invasive carcinoma of the pancreas [26].

6.3   Intraductal Papillary Mucinous Neoplasms (IPMNs)

6.3.1   Indications for Operation

IPMNs have an even greater chance of being malignant than MCNs (35). About 40 % of patients at the time of diagnosis of main-duct IPMN already have an established invasive malignancy [36, 37]. Accurate classification of IPMNs is of special clinical importance, because the risk of malignancy depends on the changes of the pancreatic ducts and its branches [38]. The risk of invasive malignancy is relatively high ($\geq$40 %) in both main-duct and mixed-duct types.

Currently, risk factors for the presence of malignancy within IPMN include [9, 36, 39]:

1. Main-duct IPMN. These IPMNs are associated with a risk of malignancy (both carcinoma in situ and invasive carcinoma) of approximately 50–60 % (and in selected situations, the risk may be as great as 92 %) [40–42]. The spectrum of atypia within an IPMN ranges from hyperplasia (adenoma) to low-grade dysplasia to high-grade dysplasia (carcinoma in situ) to invasive carcinoma. Mucinous ductal ectasia is sometimes present. Many groups have estimated a mean lag time of approximately 5 years from age at presentation of IPMN with low-grade dysplasia to the point at which it becomes an invasive carcinoma [43]. The risk of malignancy increases markedly when the main pancreatic duct is dilated more than 1 cm and when mural nodules (>1 cm) are present [36]. In contrast, the risk of some element of malignancy in branch-duct IPMN is less (6–46 %, mean 25 %) [23, 39, 41] and the risk of *invasive* carcinoma is much less [23, 42]. Factors correlating with malignancy in branch-duct IPMNs include the presence of clinical symptoms, mural nodules (especially when >2 mm), cyst size >3 cm, and coexistence of main-duct dilation [35, 39].
2. Branch-duct dilation. The presence of side branches >3 cm confers an increased risk of malignancy. The risk of malignancy in branch-duct IPMNs <2 cm was 10 % in the study by Jang et al. [44].
3. Presence of mural nodule(s).
4. Advanced age (>70 years).
5. Presence of symptoms, such as extrahepatic biliary dilation, weight loss, etc.; however, lack of symptoms does not guarantee the absence of malignancy [35].
6. Increased telomerase activity in pancreatic cystic fluid [39] and increased serum CA 19-9 levels [43].
7. A patulous papilla with leakage of mucin from the ampulla of Vater [43].

Histologic changes (atypia, dysplasia, or frank carcinoma in situ or invasive cancer) can be present concurrently in discontinuous areas throughout the pancreas, thereby raising the question of whether IPMN represents a generalized global disorder of the epithelium of the pancreatic duct or rather a localized, field defect. True multicentricity of main-duct IPMN is not common (<10 %), but in branch-duct IPMNs, multicentricity has been recognized much more frequently [35]. Multicentricity is of clinical importance for the surgeon performing pancreatectomy (see below).

Because of the overt or latent malignant potential of IPMN, operative resection is the therapy of choice in most patients with main-duct and mixed-duct IPMN, provided they are operative candidates [3, 9, 10, 14, 16, 35, 36, 38, 39, 41]. Operative therapy is more controversial with branch-duct disease alone. Analytically, a formal oncologic resection is indicated for [35, 38]:

1. Main-duct and mixed type IPMNs
2. Branch-duct IPMNs with cyst diameters of over 30 mm or cyst diameter of 10–30 mm with a mural nodule
3. Cytology-positive IPMN
4. Presence of clinical symptomatology (such as obstructive jaundice, unexplained weight loss)

Recently, a conservative management ("watchful waiting") has been proposed for selected patients with IPMNs. This approach can be considered in selected subgroups, including high-risk surgical patients if other predictors of malignancy are not present (e.g., for main-duct IPMNs, when the main pancreatic duct is smaller than 10 mm and there are no visible mural nodules). This conservative approach has been accepted with more support in selected patients with branch-duct IPMNs, given the much lesser incidence of invasive cancer in branch-duct disease [35, 36, 45, 46]. This group of patients includes asymptomatic patients with branch-duct IPMNs with cystic lesions <3 cm, no mural nodules or main-duct dilation, and no cytologic findings suspicious or positive for malignancy [35, 42, 47–49]; this approach is based on the low incidence of invasive malignancy (~2 %) in these patients, which approximates the mortality risk of a major pancreatic resection (i.e., pancreatoduodenectomy) [48]. Close follow-up using periodic cross-sectional imaging is required in these cases to detect suspicious findings suggesting a reevaluation of the situation and reassessment of the role of operative resection. The timing of surveillance is determined by cyst size [38]. Obviously, the "watchful waiting" approach is applicable only if the patient can be kept under close supervision. Tables 6.1 and 6.2 summarize the recommendations of the International Association of Pancreatology regarding optimal management of IPMNs and MCNs (Sendai 2006 and the more recent [2012] consensus guidelines) [35, 50].

6.3.2 Type of Resection

The aim of operative resection is to remove all the adenomatous or malignant ductal epithelium if possible and if reasonable to minimize the probability of recurrence in the pancreatic remnant. The basic and as yet not fully answered question is whether or

Table 6.2 International consensus conference guidelines 2012 for the management of IPMN and MCN of the pancreas

MD-IPMN
Operative resection recommended for all surgically fit patients
Segmental disease: focal anatomic pancreatic resection
Diffuse dilation of pancreatic duct, right-sided pancreatectomy (usually)
Frozen biopsy sections (resection line)
High-grade dysplasia: additional resection to negative margin
Moderate- or low-grade dysplasia: further resection controversial
Total pancreatectomy: selectively in young patients (who can manage the "apancreatic" state – diabetes and exocrine insufficiency)
BD-IPMN
Resection considered (especially in young [<65 years] patients with a cyst size >2 cm)
Patient medical comorbidities and cyst location should be taken into consideration
Conservative management with follow-up for selected patients who do not have the following risk factors of malignancy
Increasing cyst size
Mural nodules (especially when >2 mm)
Coexistence of main-duct dilatation (>7 mm)
High-grade atypia
Cytology positive for malignant cells
BD-IPMN >3 cm without risk factors predicting malignancy can be observed without immediate resection (especially in elderly frail patients)
MCN
Resection recommended for all surgically fit patients
Observation is an option in elderly or frail patients

Modified from Tanaka et al. [50]

not IPMN represents a local, clonal expansion of a site of neoplastic transformation, a localized field defect limited to a segment of the pancreas, a global abnormality in the ductal epithelium with the potential to affect all of the pancreatic ductal epithelium, or even possibly an anatomically local or global environmental stimulus, either exogenous or endogenous. If we know IPMN is a localized process, as with typical ductal cancer of the pancreas, then a focused resection of the involved anatomic region of the gland would be all that is necessary. In contrast, if IPMN is a global disorder of all the pancreatic ductal epithelium, probably then all the pancreatic duct epithelium is "at risk" of malignant transformation, and therefore, in selected individuals, a total pancreatectomy might be indicated [9]. Total pancreatectomy with its obligate apancreatic state has its own often serious problems (brittle diabetes, exocrine insufficiency) and trades one disease (IPMN) with another (the "apancreatic" state with its endocrine and exocrine deficiencies). In some patients, a total pancreatectomy may not be appropriate, especially in the elderly or the medically unsophisticated patient who will not be able to manage the endocrine and exocrine insufficiency. After total pancreatectomy, episodic hypoglycemia can be a substantive problem.

   The type of operation is determined based on the location of the IPMN and its subtype (i.e., the type of ductal distribution – main or mixed IPMN vs. branch-duct IPMN). For main-duct IPMN located in the pancreatic body/tail (10–25 % of patients) [51], distal pancreatectomy including splenectomy with frozen-section analysis of the proximal pancreatic margin is the procedure of choice [9, 39]. If the frozen section is negative for true adenomatous changes in the ductal epithelium (not reactive ductal hyperplasia), total pancreatectomy is not indicated in the absence of objective evidence that the proximal duct is involved. In contrast, when the margin is positive for invasive or noninvasive malignant IPMN, most surgeons would advocate a further "creeping" proximal pancreatic resection; if a tumor-free margin is not attainable after two further limited resections, most surgeons would proceed with total pancreatectomy, provided the patient is an appropriate candidate to manage the "disease" of the apancreatic state [10, 14, 35, 39]; obviously this discussion would have occurred preoperatively between patient and surgeon.

   When the entire pancreatic duct is diffusely dilated, the assumption is that the disease is in the pancreatic head causing obstruction by growth of the neoplasm and/ or by mucous production. Based on this assumption and provided no intraluminal or extraluminal solid mass is evident elsewhere in the duct outside the boundaries of a pancreatic head resection, a pancreatoduodenectomy is undertaken with intraoperative frozen-section analysis of the distal margin. A positive margin for adenomatous changes (again, not ductal hyperplasia) necessitates a further "creeping" distal resection, keeping in mind that IPMN may involve the pancreatic duct diffusely. If the frozen section remains positive after two attempts for further resection, total pancreatectomy should be entertained (in up to 10–20 % of patients) [35, 36, 39]. The concept of "prophylactic" total pancreatectomy is considered by most pancreatic surgeons as both unacceptably aggressive and unnecessary in most patients [52]. When evaluating the results of frozen section, it should be emphasized that the surgeon should keep in mind that even a negative margin does not assure the absence of neoplastic cells in the remaining pancreas. Unlike typical ductal carcinoma of the pancreas which is a contiguous clonal expansion and not a multicentric malignancy [53], IPMN can be a multifocal disease in up to 8–10 % of patients harboring main-duct disease with "skip" lesions, possibly indicating a generalized instability of the epithelium [35]. Intraoperative pancreatic ductoscopy to evaluate the pancreatic remnant has been tried with some success. While nodal metastases occur with invasive IPMN, at present, there is no evidence to justify an extended lymphadenectomy in the management of malignant IPMN.

   In localized branch-duct IPMNs, a segmental but formal anatomic, oncologic pancreatectomy is the favored procedure, i.e., pancreatoduodenectomy (preferentially of the pylorus-preserving type) for neoplasms located in the pancreatic head/ uncinate process, or distal pancreatectomy for body/tail lesions [39]. In multifocal branch-duct IPMN, therapeutic decisions are more difficult; ideally, these patients should be treated by total pancreatectomy, which eliminates all the foci of the disease, but the formidable and obligate long-term morbidity of total pancreatectomy must be considered seriously in this decision. A more conservative approach in this case would be an anatomic pancreatic resection removing the cystic lesions with worrisome characteristics (size >3 cm, mural nodules, abnormal cytology) and surveillance observation of the remnant gland/lesions for findings suggestive of malignancy in the remaining cystic lesions [35].

6.4 Rare Primary Pancreatic Cystic Neoplasms

6.4.1 Indications for Resection

Solid pseudopapillary neoplasms (SPNs) are usually very-low-grade, malignant neoplasms with the potential for metastatic spread, and operative resection is, therefore, recommended in all patients [54]. More than 95 % of SPNs arise in women and usually before the age of 40 years; their appearance is rather characteristic especially in a young women. Cystic neuroendocrine neoplasms are considered premalignant or malignant lesions and should be treated operatively. Typically, however, accurate preoperative identification is not possible, even using sophisticated, modern, state-of-the-art imaging and molecular techniques, and thus operative resection usually establishes the diagnosis definitively [55].

6.4.2 Type of Resection

Because of uncertainty of the diagnosis and concerns about malignancy, rare pancreatic neoplasms should be treated with a formal, anatomic pancreatic resection. Despite that theoretic concept that a more conservative approach could be acceptable in selected cases, a radical approach is preferred, especially in surgically fit patients to avoid the risk of undertreatment of a potentially curable disease [55, 56].

6.5 Comments

The overall status of the patient is a very relevant clinical consideration, which should be evaluated when deciding to resect a pancreatic cystic lesion; indeed, the risk of resection should be weighed against and not exceed the risk of concurrent or future malignancy. High-risk patients (e.g., those with severe comorbidities or advanced age) may be followed with periodic, noninvasive imaging; aggressive evaluation, including EUS with FNA cytology and analysis of cyst fluid, might not be cost-effective in these patients unless these procedures will definitely change therapy [19].

Misdiagnosing a PCN as a pancreatic pseudocyst is usually avoidable and may prove to be a serious diagnostic error. In the absence of a history of pancreatitis, the surgeon should maintain a high index of suspicion for the presence of a PCN in any patient with a cystic pancreatic lesion. Indeed, a cystic mass in the pancreas in a patient without any history of pancreatopathy should be considered a cystic neoplasm of the pancreas (most commonly, in women MCN and in men an IPMN) until proven otherwise. With time, most pseudocysts resolve spontaneously, whereas a cystic neoplasm will persist or grow. Inappropriate treatment of a MCN by cysto-gastrostomy or cystenterostomy when misdiagnosed initially as a pancreatic pseu-docyst will usually recur and may have dramatic results, which can potentially impair the patient's prognosis; this pitfall was much more common in the past, even in experienced centers [34, 57–59]. In their original report of 67 cystic pancreatic neoplasms, including 42 MCNs, Warshaw et al. found that 37 % of the neoplasms were misdiagnosed initially as pancreatic pseudocysts even when the cyst wall was "biopsied" [34]. Many of these neoplasms were treated inappropriately with cysten-terostomy procedures rather than with potentially curative resections, resulting in substantial patient morbidity and mortality. Subsequently, in a later report by the same authors, this figure decreased to 9 %, which suggests that the current height-ened awareness by surgeons, gastroenterologists, radiologists, and pathologists can decrease the number of diagnostic errors [57]. Part of the problem with the diagno-sis of MCN on intraoperative biopsy of the cyst wall is that the epithelial lining is notoriously discontinuous and may be absent in many places. Currently, clinical, epidemiologic, and imaging findings combined with the results of fluid cytology and analysis (when indicated) allow preoperative diagnosis with acceptable accu-racy; therefore, currently, this error is much less common and should be very uncommon.

6.6   Adjuvant/Neoadjuvant Therapy

6.6.1   MCN

Adjuvant therapy should at least be entertained in patients with invasive MCNs undergoing a "curative" resection, even if there are no nodal metastases and even though no formal studies have addressed the topic [9, 10, 22]. Chemotherapy should also be considered for non-resectable, advanced malignant MCNs of the pancreas [60, 61]. Although we advocate "consideration" of adjuvant therapies, the role of neoadjuvant therapy in the management of MCNs remains undefined. We need to emphasize that reliable data on the responsiveness of cystadenocarcinomas to adju-vant, neoadjuvant, and therapeutic chemotherapy or radiation therapy are lacking, because no one center has been able to generate a large enough experience with this somewhat rare subgroup of MCNs; a formal study would require a multicenter trial.

6.6.2   IPMN

As for invasive MCNs, adjuvant therapy should be considered for patients undergo-ing curative resection of invasive IPMNs [9, 14]. Due to the absence of randomized clinical trials in this topic, the type of treatment that has been adopted has been simi-lar to that for ductal adenocarcinoma, i.e., usually gemcitabine-based chemotherapy with or without radiation. In a recent study from the Johns Hopkins Hospital, 70 patients with malignant (invasive) IPMN received postoperative (adjuvant) chemo-radiotherapy, which appeared to confer a 57 % decrease in the relative risk of mortality; patients with lymph node metastases or positive margins appeared to benefit particularly from this adjuvant chemoradiation therapy after curative resection [62–64]. Caponi et al. (from Italy) in their study published a year ago concluded that adjuvant chemotherapy with gemcitabine was associated with a greater disease-free survival compared to surgery alone [64]. Other studies, however, have not suggested such an enthusiastic benefit [65]. It should be stressed that there is no level 1 or level 2 evidence addressing the topic of adjuvant chemo- or radiotherapy in IPMN.

Concerning neoadjuvant therapy in IPMN, although there is suggestive evidence that apparently unresectable neoplasms with no metastases can become resectable after combined chemoradiation therapy, experience is extremely limited and completely anecdotal, thereby precluding definite recommendations. Just as for adjuvant therapy, no good studies currently address neoadjuvant therapy. This topic also calls for a multicenter trial.

6.7 Cyst Ablation

Cyst ablation has been proposed recently as a less invasive method than pancreatic resection for the management of high-risk patients who are not ideal candidates for a major pancreatic resection. Ablation is achieved by injecting ablative agents into the cyst cavity under EUS or CT image guidance. Ethanol has been the ablative agent used most commonly, but recently paclitaxel has been added to increase the efficacy of this approach [66]. Epithelial ablation after this procedure has been documented histologically after resection of the ablated cysts [67]. Results were encouraging in lesions ranging in size from 1 to 5 cm [67, 68]. Ablation appears to achieve a decrease in size of the cystic area to <5 % of the original size in ~35 % of patients using ethanol and in 50–80 % using ethanol combined with paclitaxel [69–72]. Interestingly, Oh et al. [72] reported 52 patients who underwent EUS-guided cyst ablation using ethanol and paclitaxel; 43 of these patients were followed with complete response seen in 29 patients (67 %). More than one session of ablation may result in a significantly greater decrease in the size and surface area of the pancreatic cystic neoplasm and is associated with a greater rate of image-defined cyst resolution [73]. Cyst ablation appears to be a safe procedure with only a few post-procedure complications [67], such as pancreatitis (2–10 %), transient abdominal pain (2–20 %), fever (2 %), and intracystic bleeding (2 %) [67–73]. As expected, post-ablation morbidity is greater compared to that of EUS-guided FNA of pancreatic cyst [38].

These preliminary studies suggest that cyst ablation seems to be a promising method to be explored in the future. Currently, however, given the lack of complete ablation of the cyst epithelium, it remains an experimental approach and should be considered only as part of a clinical trial in individuals who are not operative candidates [38]. If and when this conservative strategy is adopted, both the patient and the surgeon should acknowledge and accept the risk of undertreating a potentially malignant and potentially curable neoplasm.

References

1. Salvia R, Malleo G, Marchegiani G, Pennacchio S, Paiella S, Maini M, et al. Pancreatic resections for cystic neoplasms: from the surgeon's presumption to the pathologist's reality. Surgery. 2012;152:S135–42.
2. Sahani DV, Sainani NI, Blake MA, Crippa S, Mino-Kenudson M, del-Castillo CF, et al. Prospective evaluation of reader performance on MDCT in characterization of cystic pancreatic lesions and prediction of cyst biologic aggressiveness. AJR Am J Roentgenol. 2011;197:W53–61.
3. Roggin KK, Chennat J, Oto A, et al. Pancreatic cystic neoplasm. Curr Probl Surg. 2010;47:459–510.
4. Kimura W, Moriya T, Hanada K, Abe H, Yanagisawa A, Fukushima N, Ohike N, Shimizu M, Hatori T, Fujita N, et al. Multicenter study of SCN of the Japan pancreas society: a multi-institutional study of 172 patients. Pancreas. 2012;41:380–87.
5. Abe H, Kubota K, Mori M, Miki K, Minagawa M, Noie T, Kimura W, Makuuchi M. Serous cystadenoma of the pancreas with invasive growth: benign or malignant? Am J Gastroenterol. 1998;93:1963–6.
6. Eriguchi N, Aoyagi S, Nakayama T, Hara M, Miyazaki T, Kutami R, Jimi A. Serous cystadenocarcinoma of the pancreas with liver metastases. J Hepatobil Pancreat Surg. 1998;5:467–70.
7. Khashab MA, Shin EJ, Amateau S, Canto MI, Hruban RH, Fishman EK, et al. Tumor size and location correlate with behavior of pancreatic serous cystic neoplasms. Am J Gastroenterol. 2011;106:1521–6.
8. Tseng JF, Warshaw AL, Sahani DV, Lauwers GY, Rattner DW, Fernandez-del Castillo C. Serous cystadenoma of the pancreas: tumor growth rates and recommendations for treatment. Ann Surg. 2005;242:413–19.
9. Sarr MG, Murr M, Smirk TC, et al. Primary cystic neoplasms of the pancreas: neoplastic disorders of emerging importance-current state of the art and unanswered questions. J Gastrointest Surg. 2003;7:417–28.
10. Sakorafas GH, Sarr MG. Cystic neoplasms of the pancreas; what a clinician should know. Cancer Treat Rev. 2005;31:507–35.
11. Galanis C, Zamani A, Cameron JL, et al. Resected serous cystic neoplasms of the pancreas: a review of 158 patients with recommendations for treatment. J Gastrointest Surg. 2007;11:820–26.
12. Strobel O, Z'Graggen K, Schmitz-Winnenthal FH, et al. Risk of malignancy in serous cystic neoplasms of the pancreas. Digestion. 2003;68:24–33.
13. Pyke CM, van Heerden JA, Colby TV, et al. The spectrum of serous cystadenoma of the pancreas. Ann Surg. 1992;215:132–9.
14. Sarr MG, Kendrick ML, Nagorney DM, et al. Cystic neoplasms of the pancreas. Surg Clin North Am. 2001;81:497–509.
15. Fernandez-del Castillo C, Targarona J, Thayer SP, et al. Incidental pancreatic cysts: clinicopathologic characteristics and comparison with symptomatic patients. Arch Surg. 2003;138:424–42.
16. Brugge WR, Lauwers GY, Sahani D, et al. Cystic neoplasms of the pancreas. N Engl J Med. 2004;351:1218–26.
17. Bassi C, Salvia R, Molinari E, et al. Management of 100 consecutive cases of pancreatic serous cystadenoma: wait for symptoms and see at imaging or vice versa? World J Surg. 2003;27:319–23.

18. Tseng JF. Management of serous cystadenoma of the pancreas. J Gastrointest Surg. 2008;12:408–10.
19. Sakorafas GH, Smyrniotis V, Reid-Lombardo KM, Sarr MG. Primary pancreatic cystic neoplasms revisited. Part I: serous cystic neoplasms. Surg Oncol. 2011;20:e84–92.
20. Sakorafas GH, Friess H, Balsiger MN, et al. Problems of reconstruction following pancreatoduodenectomy. Dig Surg. 2001;18:363–9.
21. Warshaw AL, Rattner DW, Fernandezdel-del Castillo C, Z'graggen K. Middle segment pancreatectomy: a novel technique for conserving pancreatic tissue. Arch Surg. 1998;133:327–31.
22. Sarr MG, Carpenter HA, Prabhakar LP, et al. Clinical and pathologic correlation of 84 mucinous cystic neoplasms of the pancreas: can one reliably differentiate benign from malignant (or premalignant) neoplasms? Ann Surg. 2000;231:205–12.
23. Katz MHG, Mortenson MM, Wang H, et al. Diagnosis and management of cystic neoplasms of the pancreas: an evidence based approach. J Am Coll Surg. 2008;207:106–20.
24. Crippa S, Salvia R, Warshaw AL, et al. Mucinous cystic neoplasm of the pancreas is not an aggressive entity: lessons from 163 resected patients. Ann Surg. 2008;247:571–79.
25. Goh BK, Yu-Meng Tan J, Chung YFA, et al. A review of mucinous cystic neoplasms of the pancreas defined by ovarian-type stroma: clinicopathological features of 344 patients. World J Surg. 2006;30:2236–45.
26. Sakorafas GH, Smyrniotis V, Reid-Lombardo KM, Sarr MG. Primary pancreatic cystic neoplasms revisited. Part II: mucinous cystic neoplasms. Surg Oncol. 2011;20:e93–101.
27. Ceppa EP, De la Fuente S, Reddy SK, et al. Defining criteria for selective operative management of pancreatic cystic lesions: does size really matter? J Gastrointest Surg. 2010;14:236–44.
28. Handrich SJ, Hough DM, Fletcher JG, Sarr MG. The natural history of the incidentally discovered small simple pancreatic cyst: long-term follow-up and clinical implications. AJR Am J Roentgenol. 2005;184:20–3.
29. Melotti G, Butturini G, Piccoli M, et al. Laparoscopic distal pancreatectomy: results on a consecutive series of 58 patients. Ann Surg. 2007;246:77–82.
30. Fernandez-del CC. Mucinous cystic neoplasms. J Gastrointest Surg. 2008;12:411–3.
31. Crippa S, Bassi C, Warshaw AL, et al. Middle pancreatectomy: indications, short- and long-term operative outcomes. Ann Surg. 2007;246:69–76.
32. Jeurnink SM, Vleggaar FP, Siersema PD. Overview of the clinical problem: Facts and current issues of mucinous cystic neoplasms of the pancreas. Dig Liver Dis. 2008;40:837–46.
33. Hutchins GF, Draganov PV. Cystic neoplasms of the pancreas: a diagnostic challenge. World J Gastroenterol. 2009;15:48–54.
34. Warshaw AL, Compton CC, Lewandrowski K, et al. Cystic tumors of the pancreas: new clinical, radiologic, and pathologic observations in 67 patients. Ann Surg. 1990;212:432–45.
35. Tanaka M, Chari S, Adsay V, Fernandez-del Castillo C, Falconi M, Shimizu M, Yamaguchi K, Yamao K, Matsuno S. International consensus guidelines for management of intraductal papillary mucinous neoplasms and mucinous cystic neoplasms of the pancreas. Pancreatology. 2006;6:17–32.
36. Sakorafas GH, Smyrniotis V, Reid-Lombardo KM, Sarr MG. Primary pancreatic cystic neoplasms revisited. Part III: intraductal papillary mucinous neoplasms. Surg Oncol. 2011;20:e109–118.
37. Adsay NV, Conlon KC, Zee SY, et al. Intraductal papillary mucinous neoplasms of the pancreas: an analysis of in situ and invasive carcinomas in 28 patients. Cancer. 2002;94:62–77.
38. Lennon AM, Wolfgang C. Cystic neoplasms of the pancreas. J Gastrointest Surg. 2013;17:645–53.
39. Farnell MB. Surgical management of intraductal papillary mucinous neoplasm (IPMN) of the pancreas. J Gastrointest Surg. 2008;12:414–6.
40. Salvia R, Fernández-del Castillo C, Bassi C, Thayer SP, Falconi M, Mantovani W, et al. Main-duct intraductal papillary mucinous neoplasms of the pancreas: clinical predictors of malignancy and long-term survival following resection. Ann Surg. 2004;239:678–87.

41. Sohn TA, Yeo CJ, Cameron JL, Hruban RH, Fukushima N, Campbell KA, Lillemoe KD. Intraductal papillary mucinous neoplasms of the pancreas: an updated experience. Ann Surg. 2004;239:788–97.
42. Sugiyama M, Izumisato Y, Abe N, et al. Predictive factors for malignancy in intraductal papillary-mucinous tumors of the pancreas. Br J Surg. 2003;90:1244–49.
43. Verbesey JE, Munson JL. Pancreatic cystic neoplasms. Surg Clin N Am. 2010;90:411–25.
44. Jang JY, Kim SW, Lee SE, et al. Treatment guidelines for branch duct type intraductal papillary mucinous neoplasms of the pancreas: when can we operate or observe? Ann Surg Oncol. 2008;15:199–205.
45. Matsumoto T, Aramaki M, Yada K, et al. Optimal management of the branch duct type IPMNs of the pancreas. J Clin Gastroenterol. 2003;36:261–5.
46. Crippa S, Fernandez-del CC. Management of intraductal papillary mucinous neoplasms. Curr Gastroenterol Rep. 2008;10:136–43.
47. Serikawa M, Sasaki T, Fujimoto Y, et al. Management of intraductal papillary mucinous neoplasm of the pancreas. Treatment strategy based on morphologic classification. J Clin Gastroenterol. 2006;40:856–62.
48. Woo SM, Ryu JK, Lee SH, et al. Branch duct IPMNs in a retrospective series of 190 patients. Br J Surg. 2009;96:405–11.
49. Rodriguez JR, Salvia R, Crippa S, et al. Branch-duct IPMNs : observations in 145 patients who underwent resection. Gastroenterology. 2007;133:72–9.
50. Tanaka M, Fernandez-del Castillo C, Adsay V, Chari S, Falconi M, Jang JY, et al. International consensus guidelines 2012 for the management of IPMN and MCN of the pancreas. Pancreatology. 2012;12:183–97.
51. Chari ST, Yadav D, Smyrk TC, et al. Study of recurrence after surgical resection of IPMN of the pancreas. Gastroenterology. 2002;123:1500–7.
52. Garcea G, Ong SL, Rajesh A, et al. Cystic lesions of the pancreas. A diagnostic and management dilemma. Pancreatol. 2008;8:236–51.
53. Tanno S, Nakano Y, Koizumi K, Sugiyama Y, Nakamura K, Sasajima J, et al. Pancreatic ductal adenocarcinoma in long-term follow-up patients with branch duct intraductal papillary mucinous neoplasms. Pancreas. 2010;39:36–40.
54. Papravramidis T, Papavramidis S. Solid pseudopapillary tumors of the pancreas: review of 718 patients reported in English literature. J Am Coll Surg. 2005;200:965–72.
55. Goh BK, Tan YM, Cheow PC, et al. Solid pseudopapillary neoplasms of the pancreas: an updated experience. J Surg Oncol. 2007;95:640–44.
56. Sakorafas GH, Smyrniotis V, Reid-Lombardo KM, Sarr MG. Primary pancreatic cystic neoplasms revisited: Part III: rare cystic neoplasms. Surg Oncol. 2012;21(3):153–63.
57. Fernandez-del Castillo C, Warshaw AL. Cystic tumors of the pancreas. Surg Clin N Am. 1995;75:1001–16.
58. Warshaw AL, Rutledge PL. Cystic tumors mistaken for pancreatic pseudocysts. Ann Surg. 1987;205:393–8.
59. Yamaguchi K, Enjoji M. Cystic neoplasms of the pancreas. Gastroenterology. 1987;92:1934–43.
60. Obayashi K, Ohwada S, Sunose Y, et al. Remarkable effect of gemcitabine-oxaliplatin (GEMOX) therapy in a patient with advanced metastatic mucinous cystic neoplasm of the pancreas. Gan To Kagaku Ryoho. 2008;35:1915–7.
61. Shimada K, Iwase K, Aono T, et al. A case of advanced mucinous cystadenocarcinoma of the pancreas with peritoneal dissemination responding to gemcitabine. Gan To Kagaku Ryoho. 2009;36:995–8.
62. Swartz MJ, Hsu CC, Pawlik TM, et al. Adjuvant chemoradiotherapy after pancreatic resection for invasive carcinoma associated with intraductal papillary mucinous neoplasm of the pancreas. Int J Radiat Oncol Biol Phys. 2010;76:839–44.
63. Schnelldorfer T, Sarr MG, Nagorney DM, et al. Experience with 208 resections for intraductal papillary mucinous neoplasm of the pancreas. Arch Surg. 2008;143:639–46.
64. Caponi S, Vasile E, Funel N, DeLio N, Campani D, Ginocchi L, et al. Adjuvant chemotherapy seems beneficial for invasive IPMN. Eur J Surg Oncol. 2013;39:396–403.

65. Turrini O, Waters JA, Schnelldorfer T, et al. Invasive intraductal papillary mucinous neoplasm: predictors of survival and role of adjuvant therapy. HPB. 2010;12(7):447–55.
66. Yoon WJ, Brugge WR. Pancreatic cystic neoplasms: diagnosis and management. Gastroenterol Clin North Am. 2012;41:103–18.
67. Gan SI, Thompson CC, Lauwers GY, Bounds BC, Brugge WR. Ethanol lavage of pancreatic cystic lesions: initial pilot study. Gastrointest Endosc. 2005;61:746–52.
68. Brugge WR. Management and outcomes of pancreatic cystic lesions. Dig Liver Dis. 2008;40:854–9.
69. Oh HC, Seo DW, Lee TY, Kim JY, Lee SS, Lee SK, et al. New treatment for cystic tumors of the pancreas: EUS-guided ethanol lavage with paclitaxel injection. Gastrointest End. 2008;67:636–42.
70. Oh HC, Seo DW, Kim SC, Yu E, Kim K, Moon SH, et al. Septated cystic tumors of the pancreas: is it possible to treat them by endoscopic ultrasonography-guided intervention? Scand J Gastroenterol. 2009;44:242–7.
71. DeWitt J, McGreevy K, Schmidt CM, Brugge WR. EUS-guided ethanol versus saline solution lavage for pancreatic cysts: a randomized, double-blind study. Gastroint Endosc. 2009;70:710–23.
72. Oh HC, Seo DW, Song TJ, Moon SH, Park do H, Soo Lee S, et al. Endoscopic ultrasonography-guided ethanol lavage with paclitaxel injection treats patients with pancreatic cysts. Gastroenterology. 2011;140:172–9.
73. DiMaio CJ, DeWitt JM, Brugge WE. Ablation of pancreatic cystic lesions: the use of multiple endoscopic ultrasound-guided ethanol lavage sessions. Pancreas. 2011;40:664–8.

Prognosis and Follow-Up

7

George H. Sakorafas, Vassileios Smyrniotis,
and Michael G. Sarr

7.1 SCN

Complete resection of SCNs ensures cure (SCN/7, 9, 24). SCNs do not recur either locally or distally after appropriate operative treatment with an R0 resection; therefore, a regular follow-up program with surveillance after complete resection is not necessary and would not be cost effective [1–3]. No adjuvant therapy is needed. For patients with SCNs treated conservatively by surveillance without resection, there are no firm guidelines about the optimal method or timing of surveillance. The interval between serial cross-sectional imaging remains controversial, but most groups recommend surveillance on an annual basis [1, 4–6], while others recommend every 2 years [6].

7.2 MCN

Complete operative resection of MCNs lacking an invasive component (i.e., benign MCNs and, more importantly, noninvasive proliferative MCNs) is a curative procedure [3, 7]). These neoplasms are solitary and do not recur either locally or distally after complete operative resection [MCN/7]. The survival of these patients is

G.H. Sakorafas, MD (✉)
Department of Surgical Oncology, Saint Savvas Cancer Hospital,
Arkadias 19-21, Athens 11526, Greece
e-mail: georgesakorafas@yahoo.com

V. Smyrniotis, MD
4th Department of Surgery, Attikon University Hospital, Chanioti 22, Athens 15452, Greece
e-mail: vsmyrniotis@hotmail.com

M.G. Sarr, MD
Department of Surgery, Mayo Clinic, 200 First Street SW, Rochester, MN 55905, USA
e-mail: sarr.michael@mayo.edu

© Springer-Verlag Italia 2015
G.H. Sakorafas et al. (eds.), *Pancreatic Cystic Neoplasms:
From Imaging to Differential Diagnosis and Management*,
DOI 10.1007/978-88-470-5708-1_7

excellent, with 100 % 5-year disease-specific survival [8]. Therefore, for patients without tissue invasion, a regular follow-up program with surveillance (using cross-sectional imaging tests) is also not necessary, thereby saving money and eliminating patient worry [4, 7–10]. One, however, must be confident in the diagnosis of MCN, being certain that the cystic lesion is not an IPMN; the presence of ovarian stroma in the pathology specimen is mandatory to exclude IPMN.

More controversial is the question of long-term survival and surveillance of the more unusual patients with MCNs with tissue invasion who undergo "curative" resection. In the past, numerous articles have claimed survival rates greater than 50 % and up to 70 % for these Grade 1 mucinous "cystadenocarcinomas" [7, 8, 11]; however, these series lumped together MCNs containing a proliferative epithelium (but without any tissue invasion) with the true cystadenocarcinomas which had tissue invasion. Occasionally, unrecognized foci of invasive carcinoma may exist within a presumably noninvasive proliferative MCN [12]; in this case, recurrence and metastases can be observed, which contrasts the absence of recurrences for "true" noninvasive MCNs after complete resection and stresses the importance of a complete histopathologic analysis of all the surface areas of a MCN [12–14]. After a careful evaluation of MCNs containing true invasive carcinoma, 5-year survival rates appear quite poor (15–35 %), albeit still somewhat better than those for typical ductal cancer of the pancreas but consistent with an aggressive malignancy [8]. The extent of invasion is the most important prognostic factor in malignant MCNs [15]. Patients with invasive MCNs require postoperative follow-up imaging, as for patients with pancreatic adenocarcinoma [4]. Some groups suggest that patients with resected malignant MCNs should be followed every 6 months regarding local recurrence and distant metastases (mainly hematogenous) using either CT or MRI [10]. The prognosis for unresectable invasive MCNs is as poor as that for unresectable pancreatic adenocarcinoma [2, 8]. The dramatic difference in prognosis for patients with noninvasive and invasive MCNs highlights the enormous importance of diagnosing and resecting noninvasive MCNs before they progress to an invasive carcinoma whenever possible [16]. Whether resection of recurrent MCN, either locally or distantly (liver, lung), is worthwhile is completely unknown.

7.3   IPMN

In IPMN, the dysplastic component may remain in situ for many years. For a single branch-duct IPMN, several studies suggest strongly that a local anatomic resection is essentially curative in most patients. In contrast, for noninvasive, main-duct IPMNs, occurrence in the remnant gland has been found with variable rates (0–20 %) [2, 9, 14], provided that the frozen-section margin is negative for adenomatous changes and the resected specimen lacks invasive IPMN. One study of patients from two large referral centers (Verona, Italy, and Boston, MA USA) maintained that after a curative resection with negative margins, recurrence is extremely rare [17]; in contrast, another large study showed an 8 % incidence of recurrence in the remnant [10]. Under these conditions, recurrence in the remnant may be due to the presence of multifocal disease [18] or to overlooked residual disease at the ductal margin. In distinct contrast, when the resection specimen contains invasive disease, even if the margins are negative, recurrent IPMN, either in the pancreatic remnant or more commonly in peripancreatic and extrapancreatic sites, occurs in 50–90 % of patients, dramatically altering prognosis and reinforcing the concept that invasive IPMN is a serious, aggressive malignancy [19, 20]. Interestingly, in the Mayo Clinic series [21] of invasive IPMN, recurrence after partial pancreatectomy (18/27; 67 %) was similar to that observed after total pancreatectomy (8/13; 62 %), suggesting no oncologic advantage to total pancreatectomy, similar in principle to ductal adenocarcinoma of the pancreas [22].

The 5-year survival after curative resection of IPMN *without* invasive cancer is >70 % in most series [21, 23]. Some reports have even suggested a 5-year survival in excess of 90 % after resection. In contrast, after resection of invasive IPMN, even with negative margins, the 5-year survival ranges from only 30 to 50 % [19–21]. Features predicting decreased survival when invasive cancer is present include lymph node metastases, vascular invasion, positive resection margins, and an invasive component measuring >2 cm [20, 24]. Invasive IPMN should be managed as an aggressive malignancy that behaves, in many respects, similar to ductal cancer of the pancreas. Overall survival, however, appears somewhat better with invasive IPMN compared to pancreatic ductal adenocarcinoma, but whether this observation is due to a stage shift with earlier diagnosis of IPMN, as shown in some studies [20], or due to a truly less aggressive tumor biology of invasive IPMN remains controversial.

Because adjuvant therapy for pancreatic ductal adenocarcinoma has been shown to improve survival, it is often recommended in the management of patients with invasive IPMN, especially in the presence of negative prognostic factors (i.e., positive lymph nodes and/or positive margins). The role of adjuvant chemotherapy or chemoradiation therapy in invasive IPMN, however, remains controversial. Interestingly, in a recent study published by Turrini et al., a notable decrease in 5-year overall survival was noted in those patients who received any adjuvant therapy [24]. In this study, re-operation for recurrence in the remnant pancreas was associated with substantial long-term survival; this aggressive surgical strategy should be considered for patients with local recurrence amenable to re-resection. In contrast, a study from Johns Hopkins suggested a survival advantage to the use of adjuvant chemoradiation therapy [25]. Obviously, this topic requires formal study (see above – ADJUVANT/NEOADJUVANT THERAPY).

Routine follow-up surveillance with noninvasive imaging appears to be relevant clinically, potentially therapeutic, and indicated in all patients with IPMNs. If recurrence occurs, selected patients may benefit from further treatment [10]. There are no established guidelines regarding the frequency or type of surveillance imaging to detect potential recurrence. A reasonable strategy for noninvasive IPMNs would be to obtain yearly follow-up with CT or MRI and then increase the interval between imaging if no changes have occurred over several years [9, 10]. For patients with noninvasive IPMN but with low- or moderate-grade dysplasia at the margin, clinical review and MRI/MRCP twice a year (if asymptomatic) have been proposed [4].

Because patients with invasive IPMN have a greater risk of recurrence, this population probably should be evaluated every 6 months with abdominal CT or MRI/MRCP [9, 10]. As noted previously, observation may well be indicated for patients with branch-duct IPMN who are asymptomatic without mural nodules in whom the main duct is not dilated (<6 mm) and the cyst size is <3 cm. The frequency of follow-up can be based on the size of the side branch IPMN: 0–1 cm, yearly; 1–2 cm, every 6–12 months; and 2–3 cm, every 3–6 months. We stress, however, that these are suggested guidelines based on the best interpretation of our current understanding. Abdominal CT, MRI/MRCP, and EUS are utilized for assessing cyst size, presence of mural nodules, and any changes in the diameter of the main duct. The interval of follow-up may be increased in duration if no change is observed during the first 2 years postoperatively [26]. The known increased risk of development of typical pancreatic ductal adenocarcinoma in patients with branch-duct IPMN should also be considered when planning follow-up in patients treated conservatively [22]. Biochemical follow-up surveillance is of little value. Tumor markers, such as serum levels of CEA and CA 19-9, have no value in the follow-up of these patients. The discovery of a pancreatic cyst/mass lesion after operative resection may be related to the presence of a postoperative contained leak, recurrence of IPMN linked to incomplete resection, a new site of IPMN, or rarely a recurrence of cystadenocarcinoma after inadequate histopathologic examination [2]. Similar considerations are pertinent after resection of main-duct IPMN. One other consideration is that dilation of the main pancreatic duct after a pancreatoduodenectomy may also be secondary to stricture at the pancreaticoenterostomy and not always from recurrent IPMN.

As mentioned above, patients with IPMN have a greater incidence (~25–30 %) of synchronous or metachronous extrapancreatic neoplasms, both benign and malignant, in other organs (including colon, rectum, stomach, lung, breast, liver, etc.), but also of typical ductal pancreatic cancer [27, 28]. This important information should be taken into consideration when scheduling both the initial evaluation and the follow-up plan of patients with IPMNs; more frequent screening colonoscopy may be warranted in these patients because of the increased frequency of colonic neoplasms [27].

7.4   Rare PCN

The prognosis of patients with SPNs is excellent after complete resection (5-year survival ~95 %) [29]. Interestingly, prognosis remains good even in patients with metastases; in one study, only 18 % of patients with metastatic disease died after a mean follow-up of 6.3 years [30]. Cross-sectional imaging every 6 months for 2 years and then every year for 5 years has been proposed for the follow-up of these patients [4]. When recurrent SPN is discovered, a very aggressive strategy of re-resection is warranted, whether the recurrence is local or distant. For patients with *cystic neuroendocrine neoplasms*, prognosis after resection is similarly good, with a 5-year survival rate of 98 % [31]. The prognosis of other rare PCNs depends on the histologic characteristics of these neoplasms; due to their rarity, no firm recommendations regarding follow-up of these patients can be proposed.

References

1. Katz MHG, Mortenson MM, Wang H, et al. Diagnosis and management of cystic neoplasms of the pancreas: an evidence based approach. J Am Coll Surg. 2008;207:106–20.
2. Sarr MG, Murr M, Smirk TC, et al. Primary cystic neoplasms of the pancreas: neoplastic disorders of emerging importance-current state of the art and unanswered questions. J Gastrointest Surg. 2003;7:417–28.
3. Sakorafas GH, Smyrniotis V, Reid-Lombardo KM, Sarr MG. Primary pancreatic cystic neoplasms revisited: part I: serous cystic neoplasms. Surg Oncol. 2011;20:84–92.
4. Lennon AM, Wolfgang C. Cystic neoplasms of the pancreas. J Gastrointest Surg. 2013;17:645–53.
5. Strobel O, Z'Graggen K, Schmitz-Winnenthal FH, et al. Risk of malignancy in serous cystic neoplasms of the pancreas. Digestion. 2003;68:24–33.
6. Tseng JF. Management of serous cystadenoma of the pancreas. J Gastrointest Surg. 2008;12:408–10.
7. Crippa S, Salvia R, Warshaw AL, et al. Mucinous cystic neoplasm of the pancreas is not an aggressive entity: lessons from 163 resected patients. Ann Surg. 2008;247:571–9.
8. Sarr MG, Carpenter HA, Prabhakar LP, et al. Clinical and pathologic correlation of 84 mucinous cystic neoplasms of the pancreas: can one reliably differentiate benign from malignant (or premalignant) neoplasms? Ann Surg. 2000;231:205–12.
9. Tanaka M, Fernandez-del Castillo C, Adsay V, Chari S, Falconi M, Jang JY, et al. International consensus guidelines 2012 for the management of IPMN and MCN of the pancreas. Pancreatology. 2012;12:183–97.
10. Tanaka M, Chari S, Adsay V, Fernandez-del Castillo C, Falconi M, Shimizu M, Yamaguchi K, Yamao K, Matsuno S. International consensus guidelines for management of intraductal papillary mucinous neoplasms and mucinous cystic neoplasms of the pancreas. Pancreatology. 2006;6:17–32.
11. Fernandez-del Castillo C. Mucinous cystic neoplasms. J Gastrointest Surg. 2008;12:411–3.
12. Wilentz RE, Albores-Saavedra J, Hruban RH. Mucinous cystic neoplasms of the pancreas. Semin Diagn Pathol. 2000;17:31–42.
13. Goh BK, Yu-Meng Tan J, Chung YFA, et al. A review of mucinous cystic neoplasms of the pancreas defined by ovarian-type stroma: clinicopathological features of 344 patients. World J Surg. 2006;30:2236–45.
14. Basturk O, Coban I, Adsay NV. Pancreatic cysts; pathologic classification, differential diagnosis, and clinical implications. Arch Pathol Lab Med. 2009;133:423–38.
15. Zamboni G, Scarpa A, Bogins G, et al. Mucinous cystic tumors of the pancreas: clinicopathological features, prognosis, and relationship to other mucinous cystic tumors. Am J Surg Pathol. 1999;23:410–22.
16. Maitra A, Fukushima N, Takaori, Hruban RH. Precursors to invasive pancreatic cancer. Adv Anat Pathol. 2005;12:81–91.
17. Salvia R, Fernandez-del Castillo C, Bassi C, et al. Main-duct intraductal papillary mucinous neoplasms of the pancreas: clinical predictors of malignancy and long-term survival following resection. Ann Surg. 2004;239:678–87.
18. Garcea G, Ong SL, Rajesh A, et al. Cystic lesions of the pancreas. A diagnostic and management dilemma. Pancreatology. 2008;8:236–51.
19. Adsay NV, Conlon KC, Zee SY, et al. Intraductal papillary mucinous neoplasms of the pancreas: an analysis of in situ and invasive carcinomas in 28 patients. Cancer. 2002;94:62–77.
20. Schnelldorfer T, Sarr MG, Nagorney DM, et al. Experience with 208 resections for intraductal papillary mucinous neoplasm of the pancreas. Arch Surg. 2008;143:639–46.

21. Chari ST, Yadav D, Smyrk TC, et al. Study of recurrence after surgical resection of IPMN of the pancreas. Gastroenterology. 2002;123:1500–7.
22. Tanno S, Nakano Y, Koizumi K, Sugiyama Y, Nakamura K, Sasajima J, et al. Pancreatic ductal adenocarcinoma in long-term follow-up patients with branch duct intraductal papillary mucinous neoplasms. Pancreas. 2010;39:36–40.
23. Jang JY, Kim SW, Lee SE, et al. Treatment guidelines for branch duct type intraductal papillary mucinous neoplasms of the pancreas: when can we operate or observe? Ann Surg Oncol. 2008;15:199–205.
24. Turrini O, Waters JA, Schnelldorfer T, Lillemoe KD, Yiannoutsos CT, Farnell MB, Sarr MG, Schmidt CM. Invasive intraductal papillary mucinous neoplasm; predictors of survival and role of adjuvant therapy. HPB. 2010;12:447–55.
25. Swartz MJ, Hsu CC, Pawlik TM, et al. Adjuvant chemoradiotherapy after pancreatic resection for invasive carcinoma associated with intraductal papillary mucinous neoplasm of the pancreas. Int J Radiat Oncol Biol Phys. 2010;76:839–44.
26. Farnell MB. Surgical management of intraductal papillary mucinous neoplasm (IPMN) of the pancreas. J Gastrointest Surg. 2008;12:414–6.
27. Reid-Lombardo KM, Mathis KL, Wood CM, et al. Frequency of extrapancreatic neoplasms in intraductal papillary mucinous neoplasm of the pancreas: implications for management. Ann Surg. 2010;251:64–9.
28. Calculli L, Pezzilli R, Brindisi C, et al. Pancreatic and extrapancreatic lesions in patients with intraductal papillary mucinous neoplasms of the pancreas; a single-centre experience. Radiol Med. 2010;115:442–52.
29. Papavramidis T, Papavramidis S. Solid pseudopapillary tumors of the pancreas: review of 718 patients reported in English literature. J Am Coll Surg. 2005;200:965–72.
30. Horisawa M, Niinomi N, Sato T, Yokoi S, Oda K, Ichikawa M, et al. Frantz's tumor (solid and cystic tumor of the pancreas) with liver metastasis: successful treatment and long-term follow-up. J Ped Surg. 1995;30:724–6.
31. Valsangkar N, Morales-Oyarvide V, Thayer S, Ferrone C, Wargo J, Warshaw A, et al. 851 resected cystic tumors of the pancreas: a 33-year experience at the Massachusetts General Hospital. Surgery. 2012;152(3 Suppl 1):S4–12.